THE
SMOOTH
RIVER

E FRONT LINE

THE
SMOOTH
RIVER

Finding Inspiration
and Exquisite Beauty
during Terminal Illness

Foreword by Lynne Holden, MD

Richard S. Cohen

Smooth River® is a trademark of Smooth River, Inc.
Published by Smooth River, Inc.

For information about this title or to order other books and/or electronic media, contact the publisher:

Smooth River, Inc.
www.smoothriver.org
office@smoothriver.org

ISBN: 978-1-7375034-0-8

Published in the United States of America

Those who learned to know death, rather than to fear and fight it, become our teachers about life.

—Elisabeth Kübler-Ross

To all those touched by terminal illness and all those who carry on the legacies of their fallen loved ones . . . and to Marcia and the fallen, who continue to live within us.

Contents

Foreword

For the past twenty-five years, I have practiced medicine at one of the busiest emergency departments at one of the largest urban hospitals in the country. My workplace is in the Bronx, New York, at Montefiore Medical Center (Moses Campus), where I never know who will pass through the emergency department doors, sometimes limping on crutches, sometimes draped over companions, sometimes in a wheelchair, sometimes on an ambulance stretcher. Even though I meet the majority of patients for the first time in an emergency setting, we have to connect. Lives depend on it! I never know what is afflicting them. I take all patients as they come, with any problem you can think of: allergic reactions, heart attacks, strokes, appendicitis, drug overdoses, respiratory problems, delirium, sepsis, trauma, and injuries of all sorts. Whatever the problem, as the attending physician, I have to lead the team and set the tone.

As an emergency medicine doctor, I carefully and quickly assess the urgent or emergent condition to stabilize and treat the patient or refer them to specialists who might be able to do so. Since the age of six, I wanted to become a doctor to heal—to help patients have the very best outcome possible. This is often the case. However, I am also confronted with patients in dire straits where the prognosis is not good. I still cringe and search for the right things to say when I have to break bad news to a patient and his or her family, especially when it's unexpected.

My colleagues and I thought we had seen it all until the coronavirus pandemic hit. And our hospital was hit hard. The sheer volume of patients struck by this deadly disease, funneling in rapid succession through the emergency department into the intensive care unit or newly converted patient care areas, was almost overwhelming. I'm still trying to make sense of the many patients whose lives were cut short: rushes of humanity draped from head to toe in masks, gowns, goggles, and respiratory gear, seeking to breathe. None of these barriers could hide the fear and desperation in their eyes, often the only channel we providers had to connect with these otherwise faceless strangers. Under quarantine conditions, their families were forced to send love and support at a distance. I'm still trying to remember the individuality of each person touched by this virulent virus and learning to be a better communicator when it comes to delivering bad news.

But the shock of receiving bad news still leaves me numb. And so it was when Richard told me in September 2019 that, out of the blue, Marcia had been diagnosed with stage 4 pancreatic cancer. My husband and I have known

Richard and Marcia for years. They supported our nonprofit, Mentoring in Medicine, Inc., which helps underprivileged students pursue health-care careers. Marcia was a powerhouse! She was the public relations guru in crisis management to the rich and famous at one of the most prominent PR firms in the country. And now she had to deal with the crisis of a lifetime.

My husband and I visited Marcia during her illness and could not shake that shock of something so bad happening to someone so good. Our hearts went out to her, and we just wanted to do something to help. However, we were struck by the grit, grace, and survival instincts that she and Richard displayed. They inspired courage in accepting an inconceivable reality, seeking to optimize a bad situation they—and science—had no control over. When we came by to lift Richard and Marcia up, they, in turn, lifted us.

And so, while I mourn the loss of Marcia, I am grateful to her for her clarity and insight. Her journey paved the way for this very moving, insightful book. *The Smooth River* tugged at my heart as a human and my mind as a professional. It gave me the perspective that was tested during the pandemic. There are important lessons for patients and health-care professionals alike. While medical school and residency training are vital, *The Smooth River* makes clear that we doctors have a lot to learn from our patients.

This book has changed the way I practice. I now try harder to see every patient beyond his or her medical problem. I look them in the eye and seek to express empathy for their circumstances. While the time that one spends with

patients in the emergency department is limited by neces-
sity, creating rapport, managing their expectations, and
appreciating their broader lives remain important to good
care. If allowed by the patient, family members can become
an integral part of the experience. I teach my residents and
medical students that each patient matters, whatever the
medical outcome may be.

The Smooth River has sensitized me to be more realistic,
straightforward, and honest with patients and their families
about medical prospects. While delivering a jarring message can be challenging, it also can be enlightening. It can
shed light on a precarious situation, spur fruitful discussion, and create a thoughtful, strategic plan of action. I've
come to realize that doctors can make an invaluable impact
helping patients prepare for possible closure and making
the most of their remaining time. Physicians don't train for
this, but avoiding the elephant in the room helps no one.
We should be looking out for a patient's best interests, and
sometimes, we need to unlock the psychological tumblers
in ourselves to figure out how best to communicate with
the people we treat.

Derived from Marcia's clarity and *The Smooth River*'s wisdom, I've developed a simple rule of thumb: I put myself in
the shoes of my patient. How would I like to be treated? It
doesn't take a lot more time to shed our defense mechanisms
and treat patients as fellow humans. Like life, the quality of
time we spend with patients and others is more important
than the quantity.

The Smooth River lifted a weight for me. It helped free me to see the entire patient, and it empowered me to encourage them to visualize their lives beyond their medical condition. There is a lot to learn from these pages. For all of us.

—Lynne Holden, MD

Professor, Emergency Medicine, Albert Einstein College of Medicine;

Vice-Chair, Diversity and Inclusion and Attending Physician, Department of Emergency Medicine, Albert Einstein College of Medicine;

President, Mentoring in Medicine, Inc.

Prologue

This book was conceived, developed, and written to help other people who have entered the turbulent world of life-threatening illness. Those undergoing other serious challenges may also find inspiration within these pages.

Although this book is about a patient and her husband and family, it is not a memoir like the many beautiful stories written by or about patients who have been beset by serious illness. *The Smooth River* provides a direct window into one family's 160-day experience with stage 4 pancreatic cancer and is offered as a gentle invitation for readers to derive their own insights into this deeply personal journey and to apply them to their own turbulent circumstances.

While the book provides advice, it is a narrative that first tells the story of how my wife and I discovered beauty within crisis. It is not a guide in the traditional sense. Its advice is intentionally inferential versus overtly prescriptive as the reader navigates the pivotal moments of our intense, five-month adventure. But by being based on frontline experience, it does, however, suggest information, guidance, and approaches that can be personalized for a wide spectrum of readers. Summarized Smooth River lessons are provided at the end. Additional resources are offered in the appendices and on the Smooth River website: www.smoothriver.org.

Contracting a terminal illness and the roller coaster one gets strapped into while dealing with it are not unique. Cancer, heart disease, amyotrophic lateral sclerosis (ALS), Alzheimer's disease, and other deadly ailments afflict millions of people and force them through all sorts of life-altering gyrations. The point of this book is not to compare our medical ride with others, but rather to describe our reaction to and management of a fatal predicament in the hope that others may gain some inspiration, peace, and new ways of thinking in regard to their own plight.

While circumstances will vary considerably from patient to patient, when mortal crisis strikes, it strips away our protective layers and differences. All of us are then left with the same dilemma—making sense of life and death.

The Smooth River was not written by a medical or "art of dying well" expert but by a regular person—a peer who, with his wife, found themselves on the firing line and needed to think and act quickly and creatively. Our experience was derived under extreme pressure and spawned a discerning Medical Plan that could absorb the shocks of disappointment as my wife's health steadily deteriorated and a Life Plan whose DNA was peace, calm, and composure for ourselves and those surrounding us.

The names of some individuals and medical institutions have been changed in keeping with the constructive spirit and delicate nature of this book. However, day counts of important events along our journey are sprinkled throughout to provide a chronology.

Normalizing end-of-life matters—and dispelling societal distortions that avoid addressing them—are critically important not just for the seriously ill and the elderly, but for everyone. Bright lights need to be shined on making life more meaningful during our final months and years . . . and well before.

I wish I had known decades ago what I know now. Hopefully, the lessons I have learned in traveling to the slippery edges where life meets death can benefit others earlier in their journeys. We need not wait for a life-threatening event to reach a deeper appreciation of who and what is in front of us now.

1. The Suddenness of It All

Life turns on a dime. Sometimes towards us,
but more often it spins away, flirting and flashing as it goes.
~Stephen King

Marcia didn't know quite what to make of the trip we were about to go on. We had been married for thirty-seven years and had been on many adventures together. But none like this.

It was the last week in June 2019, and we were about to be taken around Israel, Jordan, and the West Bank by a Muslim Palestinian woman Marcia had never met. I had met Rahima, a married PhD and mother of four, only once. It was eighteen months earlier in Briarcliff Manor, New York, during a talk she was giving about issues Muslim women have within Muslim communities in Israel. Having conducted interfaith relations for years and being fascinated by people different than me, I introduced myself to her before her presentation. Although fluent in Hebrew and Arabic, she was unsure of her English and in unfamiliar surroundings—a suburban New York City synagogue—so I hoped to make her comfortable and provide a friendly connection. She was smart, funny, and balanced, rooted in academic rigor, not rancor. Sometimes, you can tell in an instant when you click with someone: eyes light up, facial muscles soften, and a smile emerges. For more than a year after her talk, while we texted via WhatsApp, Rahima repeated warm invitations for Marcia and me to visit her so she could immerse us in Arab culture. Her good-natured persistence eventually won us over, and off we went.

Marcia and I arranged for our flight to arrive in the late afternoon on Friday, June 28, so that we could immediately go to our modest hotel, shower, have an early dinner by ourselves, and recuperate from the long flight. Rahima would have none of that. She was so excited that we had come that she met us at Ben Gurion Airport. Sharing a kindhearted demeanor, Rahima and Marcia bonded as soon as they met in the terminal.

On the walk to her car, Rahima asked us to stop; took a deep, nervous breath; and squared off to face us, clearly looking for the right words for whatever it was she wanted to say. After a few moments of staring at us in silence, she finally let out what she had been holding in for the past few months: how greatly moved and honored she was that we trusted her with this trip even though we really didn't know her.

And so began a life-changing journey. For the next two inseparable weeks, she took us deep into Arab and Druze cultures, taking care of all the arrangements and, despite my objections, virtually all the meals. It was part of ancient Arab hospitality.

When we returned to New York in mid-July, Marcia and I tried to get our minds around the immensity of the trip. The experience had overwhelmed us and kindled relationships with Palestinian and Jewish change agents that we could build upon in seeking to bridge gaps in the Middle East in our own modest way. Set against this backdrop, the mild stomach pain Marcia experienced upon our return seemed unimportant. When after a few days it didn't go away, she called a gastroenterologist, probably worried she might come across as a hypochondriac.

That was how it started.

My wife was Marcia Horowitz. She spent her entire professional life as a crisis manager advising high-profile clients and organizations. On September 3, 2019, she found herself in one crisis even she couldn't navigate. A CT scan revealed that she had stage 4 pancreatic cancer, considered the most lethal cancer. It has the lowest survival rate and one of the shortest life expectancies of all cancers: a median of three to six months after diagnosis, by some accounts. Pancreatic cancer is the third-leading cause of cancer-related deaths in the United States, behind lung and colorectal cancer. In 2020, an estimated 57,600 new cases of pancreatic cancer were diagnosed in the United States, and 47,050 people will die from the disease. Because its symptoms are hard to discern and there are no effective screening tests, a majority of patients with pancreatic cancer (like some other cancers) are first diagnosed in stage 4, after it has spread beyond the pancreas and becomes inoperable. Marcia's had invaded her liver and abdominal lining.

On February 10, 2020, 160 days after her diagnosis and a month after her sixty-eighth birthday, Marcia passed away in her sleep, at peace with herself, her family, and the world around her.

Through it all, this one patient and her family met short-term terminal illness head-on—with vigor and strength, deploying all they and medicine had to offer. But in contrast with prevailing expectations, we developed a far more expansive view of what strength means in response to life-threatening hardship. We faced the entire experience with composure and clarity by adapting to the new reality, appreciating the miracles of the mundane, and discovering the intense beauty and love that, after reasonable medical measures had failed, the process of dying offered. We called this the Smooth River. This proved to be a way of thinking that was so uplifting and natural that it continues to guide and nourish my family through the voids of grief, and will inspire us for the rest of our lives. Our five-month experience was so distinct and powerful that I've been encouraged to share it in an effort to help other individuals and families encountering terminal illness, life-threatening hardship, or serious challenges of any nature, especially where life's fuse is short.

There are books, articles, and blog posts profiling so-called success stories in managing cancer, even stage 4 metastatic cancer. There are inspiring stories of those who experienced a remission of the disease for long periods of time. These writings provide hope and motivation to those afflicted and are critically important in informing patients and clinicians of possible outcomes and in defying the odds. The problem is that these writings do not speak for huge patient populations battling advanced, aggressive cancer or other diseases likely to end their lives within a compressed time period. They don't speak to the large number of patients like Marcia who were given a bleak prognosis, where treatment success is unlikely, and the end is in sight. For these patients, the prevailing view is gloomy, and these writings offer little guidance. One can almost feel shunned and on your own because you don't represent a cancer "victory." This was unacceptable to Marcia and me. We were determined to chart our own course through the storm, set our own tone, and find our own light.

Marcia was a press communications pioneer, having worked for decades alongside public relations legend Howard Rubenstein (who himself passed away in December 2020 at the age of eighty-eight). She trained scores of employees, headed three practices, and defused hundreds of problems for clients. She was an example of a kind, organized, modest, and highly effective professional rising to the top and becoming respected by virtually everyone she touched. However serious the problem, Marcia always found calm within the storm and provided a clear, forthright, and balanced approach to convey to the press and the public. She had an intuitive knack for reducing very complex matters to a digestible and straight-forward narrative that resonated with clients under severe pressure—public figures and celebrities, large companies, law firms, private equity funds, universities, prestigious prep schools, and nonprofits. Her common sense and press-savvy insights made her indispensable to them. Clients knew she had their back, not her own. She had a quiet charisma and authenticity that made people feel safe.

Marcia was on the speed dial of top executives at leading hospitals who sought her magic touch in times of turmoil. She understood the health-care system well and knew the shortest distance between two points, despite layers of convention and complexity that might obscure the picture.

In all other aspects of her life, Marcia was well loved, sincere, and unpretentious. She was so humble that many people outside of work had little idea what she had accomplished professionally or how effectively and quietly she moved behind the headlines they were reading. She was tolerant of imperfections in herself and others and lived in the big picture. And first in the big picture was her family—our two sons, daughter-in-law, toddler grandson, and me. She had her priorities straight and would not be distracted by clutter, spin, or BS.

Soon after the diagnosis, Marcia applied this same clear-headed approach to dealing with her cancer, her treatment, and the possibility of dying. Her mindset, adopted by me and our family, was one of transparency, serenity, and adjusting to a new normal. She wanted to see her life as full, not cut short by tragedy. She took on the cancer aggressively with months of punishing chemo, twice-daily subcutaneous injections of investigational medications, natural remedies prescribed by integrative medicine specialists, and unconventional compounds we identified and used under our oncologist's supervision (such as the human form of an antiparasitic medication used for dogs). Throughout, Marcia accepted her grim circumstances with grit, grace, and humor. She had the mettle to want to understand what many people avoid: the probability of imminent death.

This supple, expansive Smooth River attitude was an incomparable gift. Marcia loved being around water. The purifying, peaceful properties of flowing water complemented her clear, direct, and unencumbered attitude toward life. The Smooth River way of thinking was so vital that we wouldn't let anything disrupt it—not the devastating march of pancreatic cancer, not the strongest chemos and their failures to work, not the frequent episodes of severe pain, not how those around us might have expected us to think or act, and not dying itself. She and I spoke about everything—her physical pain, her concerns and anxieties, her wishes. We discussed her broken heart that we would not grow old together; that she would not see her children, daughter-in-law, and grandson ripen; and that, as Marcia's condition precipitously declined, she wouldn't experience the upcoming birth of her granddaughter (Mara Sophia, born five months after she passed and who is named in her memory). Marcia needed to clear her mind, to understand the shape of her earthly time, and to leave this world in peace, with no unfinished business or words unspoken. It would be a calm float through white waters.

Although we came up with the term *Smooth River* as a metaphor for the doctors and nurses to convey that we wanted a well-ordered and tranquil ending, this perspective permeated our entire experience. We had no idea how critical this thinking would be in helping us transition from the shock of her diagnosis, to the ups and downs of her treatment and care, to her final days and passing, and then in carrying our family through the funeral, burial, and life without her. Smooth River thinking—a moving, living, transcendent outlook, soft and strong, liquid and doable, inspirational and nourishing—has provided us with safe-harbor guidance to make her life and ours a blessing.

As Marcia's husband, I coordinated her Medical Plan and collaborated with her in setting our Life Plan. Her wishes were for clarity, practicality, directness, and relief from pain so that her remaining time could be filled with peace, dignity, and love unburdened by discomfort. With medical treatment outcomes uncertain and time shrinking, every day was precious.

Our story, then, is far different from the frenetic, fevered atmosphere experienced by many terminally ill patients and their families that leaves them exhausted and unsatisfied.

Born in a slow-motion, five-month cauldron, Smooth River thinking can inspire and guide other terminally ill patients and their families through their journeys too. Hopefully it will give voice to all patients in the throes of disease—those who had treatments they deem successful and those who did not, those whose lives were extended and those whose were not.

The wide expanse of the Smooth River extends well beyond the ill. We will all die one way or another, and we all confront pressures that test our willpower. The lessons are universal.

2. The Problem: The Conventional Saying "Attitude Is Everything" Is Not Everything

Cancer is not a game of winners and losers.
If you live you "win" and if you die you "lose"?
How inappropriate is that?
~Michael A. Wosnick, retired cancer researcher

Many say that in dealing with cancer, attitude is everything. But what they mostly mean is a "fight," "win," and "beat the cancer" attitude. While a positive attitude and strong will to live can be great motivators, in many dire situations, the conventional "attitude is everything" meaning is too limited. It can be deceptive and unreal. This distortion is part of an overexpressed cultural viewpoint that likens disease management to a sport or battle involving "never giving up," "going down swinging," and "being tough in the face of adversity." It is an outgrowth of an unwillingness to confront the troubling truths about certain illnesses and the finite nature of life.

Obviously, curing a patient of any disease is a wonderful goal. But for many terminal diseases, there are no reliable treatments. There are no cures. A narrow focus on overcoming a powerful illness, without properly accounting for the full dimension of a patient's life, can involve artificial reference points and false hope measured against an unmeetable standard of beating the disorder.

Our customary blind spots regarding terminal disease can even get transmuted into putting an impossible and inappropriate burden on the patient to battle a condition for which medicine has no solution. The result is that patients can be looked down upon for not attaining an unattainable threshold: "winning." Placing undue weight on a winning attitude and "beating the thing," without understanding the realities of serious illness and the bigger picture of a patient's life, can create stigmas and even blame of the patient for contracting the illness, not defeating it, and not delivering a Hollywood happy ending for everyone.[1]

In relation to the death of Congressman John Lewis from stage 4 pancreatic cancer, oncology surgeon Mary Dillhoff said, "I really despise the metaphor of fighting a battle because I see people every day who are trying as hard as they can to live with this diagnosis. You can try to use your remaining time better, but I don't like people to think that if they just fight

---

1 Marie Ennis-O'Connor, "Words Matter: Why Cancer Isn't a Game of Winners or Losers," *Patient Empowerment Network,* April 24, 2019, https://powerfulpatients. org/2019/04/24/words-matter-why-cancer-isnt-a-game-of-winners-or-losers/.

hard enough, this is something they can beat. This is an evil cancer, and it's going to do what it does."[2]

Critical of news accounts characterizing movie critic Roger Ebert's death as having "lost his battle with cancer," retired cancer researcher Michael A. Wosnik wrote, "For those who ultimately die from a cancer, the idea that they have 'lost' a battle implies to me that if they had just done SOMETHING else differently then maybe they might have 'won.' The use of the word 'lose' is like a zero-sum game to me: if someone or something 'loses' then that means that someone or something else 'wins' . . . Roger Ebert did not lose his battle with cancer. He lived graciously and courageously with it until the very end. In many, many ways, by inspiring and teaching us, he won his battle in other very important ways."[3]

In the broader culture, we tend to reward fighters and disparage people whom we think give up. Even well-intentioned organizations promote those whom they classify as "success stories," leaving out and implicitly labeling as failures a great many patients for whom medical remedies did not work. While positive messaging can encourage patients to take an active role in their care, maintain a positive outlook, and partake in reasonable treatments, it's not the full picture. A patient's life and remaining time are bigger than any medical treatment or outcome and should not be graded by a clinical success

2 James Hamblin, "John Lewis and the Fight That Can't Be Won," *The Atlantic*, December 31, 2019, https://www.theatlantic.com/health/archive/2019/12/lewis-fight/604249/?gclid=CjwKCAjwiOv7BRBREiwAXHbv3AtN9pC-j7vll0q-4wLSt8qqNSTKCKKKY8Yx76YkrHrCawXj6mg6TjxoCMqUQAvD_BwE.
3 Michael A. Wosnick, "When Dealing with Cancer, 'Lost Battle' Language Is Inappropriate," *Healthy Debate*, April 15, 2013, https://healthydebate.ca/opinions/when-dealing-with-cancer-lost-battle-language-is-inappropriate/.

or failure or the patients' performance based on contorted expectations of how they should act or feel.

Virtually all clinicians say they are interested in a patient's quality of life, but this can become blurry if a medical intervention is recommended without fully understanding what quality of life means to the patient once fully informed of his or her prospects. In an effort to create an aura of optimism, the prospect of death is often avoided or given short shrift.

Decades ago, Elisabeth Kübler-Ross's groundbreaking work, *On Death & Dying: What the Dying Have to Teach Doctors, Nurses, Clergy & Their Families*, opened a public conversation on what was considered a taboo subject: the process of dying and the needs of terminally ill patients. She paved the way for the fields of hospice care and palliative medicine to advance the interests of the whole patient and his or her quality of life. Yet, even today, death remains a difficult subject for many professionals and laymen, and discussing its probability can be seen as a sign of giving up. If death as a reasonable likelihood is not given sufficient weight, patients and their families can be lulled into pursuing treatments that do more harm than good, heighten anxiety levels, and set everyone up for heartbreaking disappointment if the treatments do not work as expected.

Marcia yearned for visibility into the future, even though it was uncertain. Sometimes, a patient's premonitions about dying can be regarded as pessimism. Sometimes, only the patient can feel the end nearing. Sometimes, that sense is hard to articulate. Marcia felt it, though. She was a great sport; she tried everything. But she knew something no one else knew. I could see it in her eyes, in her whole demeanor.

Marcia and I braced ourselves for whatever the future held. We understood that her situation was tenuous and readied ourselves for all possible outcomes. Our oncologists were open with us, but many terminally ill patients have a different experience. Reflecting a rampant societal dilemma, large numbers of patients and their families are not properly prepared for death and are caught off guard with little time to make tangible and intangible arrangements for, and come to terms with, the end.

It is well documented that the medical profession generally is focused on curing disease and solving problems but is less adept at treating the patient as distinct from his or her medical condition. And worse yet is the squeamishness many doctors have in addressing negative medical outcomes, especially the prospects of dying. As palliative care expert Dr. Anthony Back noted in an article: "Robust research shows that doctors are notoriously bad at delivering life-altering news."[4]

Impending death can be perceived by physicians that they have failed. In their poignant memoir, *Conversations at Midnight: Coming to Terms with Dying and Death*, Kay and Herbert Kramer wrote in relation to the doctors' inability to cope with the imminent death of Herbert's first wife: "It was as if her failure to be cured was an affront to their profession, the result of some moral weakness in her. This almost universal inability to come to terms with the blunt fact of her death forced her to be the comforter, to get them [the doctors] off

4 JoNel Aleccia, "Never Say 'Die': Why So Many Doctors Won't Break Bad News," *KHN*, June 12, 2019, https://khn.org/news/never-say-die-why-so-many-doctors-wont-break-bad-news/.

the hook by demonstrating her acceptance of the presence of death." The Kramers went on to say, "Too often, in the presence of a dying person, the approach of death is never mentioned. Conversation is sanitized and the end itself, whatever it is the end of, is treated as some awful obscenity."

At the most critical moment—when patients may not know their prospects and the pros and cons of various treatments or may be in denial when they desperately need clarity—some doctors succumb to their own weaknesses and shirk what may be the most important conversation of a patient's life. Failing to address the prospects of dying can lead to unnecessary, costly, and unwanted procedures and engender emotional turmoil and confusion for everyone involved. Avoidance denies the patient the empowering right to live his or her remaining time as he or she chooses.

Study after study demonstrates the discomfort many doctors have in speaking with their patients about life beyond the disease. One study published in the *Journal of Clinical Oncology* in 2016 revealed that only 5 percent of cancer patients with less than six months to live had an accurate understanding of their illness, and 38 percent couldn't remember speaking to their doctor about their life expectancy. In a 2012 study published in *The New England Journal of Medicine*, 69 percent of patients with metastatic lung cancer and 81 percent of people with advanced colorectal cancer thought they could still be cured, although both conditions are generally considered fatal.

A Kaiser Healthcare News article summarized the problem: "In some cases, oncologists fail to tell patients how long they have to live. In others, patients are clearly told their prognosis, but are too overwhelmed to absorb the information. Some doctors and patients enter into an implicit agreement to avoid talking about dying, a pact that researchers have described as 'necessary collusion.'"[5]

Holly Prigerson, a radiation oncologist researching the problem, remarked, "We were astonished to learn that only 5 percent of the 178 terminally ill patients sampled had sufficient knowledge about their illness to make informed decisions about their care."[6]

The cultural forces that shun end-of-life discussions by both doctors and patients can lead to unfounded optimism and gross errors in forecasting how long a patient has to live. Another study, of 468 terminally ill cancer patients, found only 20 percent of the doctors involved accurately predicted how long patients would survive. Most estimated that patients would live five times longer than they did.[7]

Part of the solution of normalizing end-of-life considerations is to include them in the education curriculum for health-care professionals. As Dr. Atul Gawande said in his seminal book, *Being Mortal: Medicine and What Matters in the End*: "I learned about a lot of things in medical school, but mortality wasn't one of them . . . Our textbooks had almost nothing

5 Liz Szabo, "'How Long Have I Got, Doc?' Why Many Cancer Patients Don't Have Answers," *KHN*, June 12, 2017, https://khn.org/news/how-long -have-i-got-doc-why-many-cancer-patients-dont-have-answers/.

6 VOA News, "Only 5% of Terminally Ill Cancer Patients Fully Understand Prognosis," *Voice of America*, May 24, 2016, https://www.voanews.com/science-health/ only-5-terminally-ill-cancer-patients-fully-understand-prognosis.

7 Nicholas A. Christakis and Elizabeth B. Lamont, "Extent and Determinants of Error in Doctors' Prognoses in Terminally Ill Patients: Prospective Cohort Study," *The BMJ*, February 19, 2000, https://www.ncbi.nlm.nih.gov/pmc/articles/PMC27288/ also http://chronicle.uchicago.edu/000302/ill.shtml.

on aging or frailty or death. How the process unfolds, how people experience the end of their lives, and how it affects those around them seemed beside the point. The way we saw it . . . the purpose of medical schooling was to teach how to save lives, not how to tend to their demise."

There are an increasing number of experts stressing the importance of better educating health-care workers to have conversations with terminally ill patients about death and dying. But health-care professionals need not wait for any formal training to exercise compassion and bring out their humanity in dealing with a dying patient. All they need to do is take a deep breath and be present with the patient and family. Medical care would be advanced by widening the "fight the cancer" and "got to find a cure" perspectives to include more empathy for patients by envisioning how they would like to be treated. While many patients may not want to come to terms with the upsetting realities, providers should not shy away from uncomfortable end-of-life conversations, forcing the patient to fend for him- or herself. This is why the fields of palliative medicine, hospice, and psychology have so much to offer in embracing a more open, solicitous approach to death and dying and "full patient" care.

By caring *about* patients—not just *for* them—professionals can give them the dignity they crave and draw the satisfaction that drove them to careers to help those in need. So much good comes from just looking a patient in the eye and speaking from the heart as well as the mind. A modern version of the Hippocratic Oath includes the following: "I will remember that there is art to medicine as well as science, and that warmth, sympathy, and understanding may outweigh the surgeon's knife or the chemist's drug."[8]

Managing difficult circumstances by softening long-held preconceptions and adjusting to uncomfortable realities go to the heart of the Smooth River approach.

---

8 William C. Shiel Jr., MD, FACP, FACR, "Medical Definition of Hippocratic Oath," *MedicineNet*, https://www.medicinenet.com/script/main/art.asp?articlekey=20909.

3. The Attitude That Is Everything: The Smooth River

The question is not how to get cured, but how to live.
~Joseph Conrad

Attitude *is* everything, but the attitude Marcia and I adopted was very different from the conventional "fight the cancer" mode that is prominent in our culture. We were not going to let distorted notions define whether we won or lost, whether we were successful or not. No matter what, after gaining a good understanding of our medical options and exercising thoughtful decision-making, our experience would be on our terms. This approach formed the headwaters of the Smooth River. They would quickly advance from streamlet strands of thought into the mature, more potent flow of an all-encompassing perspective as we progressed through Marcia's illness.

It is shocking to hear a diagnosis of stage 4 pancreatic cancer, one of the worst possible cancers with the shortest time for survival. We knew instantly our lives would radically change, and we would enter a turbulent world where all the bearings that are part of a normal life were no longer there. While it took some time to absorb the shock and adjust to our new world, we reached an understanding that whatever came along, we would not accept free fall. That was not our nature. We wanted order, not chaos. We wanted some element of control, certainly over how we saw things. We wanted to maintain the integrity, discipline, and thinking that had always shaped our lives. We did not want to be subjected to clichés, pressures, or pity—the banal expectations that society applies to those with cancer, especially terminal cancer.

We sought out and took advice from the best medical experts we could find, but not blindly. Being a crisis management expert, Marcia did what she always did—she digested the information and resources we both gathered and, with my help, intuitively devised a way of evaluating her disease, managing it with all reasonable measures, and living with it, all in the broader context of her entire life. We sought candid assessments about her prognosis and life expectancy and unpacked the nuanced responses doctors gave us that sought to balance optimism and realism. We wanted unvarnished information so we could develop our own response and make our decisions on a sensible and sound basis.

Our attitude was to adjust to our new circumstances: a severely contracted world anchored on survival that also recognized the prospect of death in the near future. We would fight the cancer, but we would do so mindfully. We kept faith in medicine's capacity to restore and hoped that high-octane chemo would restrain the disease, ease Marcia's pain, and extend her life with quality. We were upbeat about achieving a good medical outcome but steeled ourselves for all eventualities. This was how the Smooth River approach took shape.

All cancer is terrible; all terminal illness is. And no one is immune. But while we may not be able to control how, if, or when we get it; how it behaves; or how effective treatment will be, we do have a choice. We can ignore reality, put on blinders, and succumb to the typical, seductive drumbeat to cheer up patients and avoid speaking about the possibility of death. Or we can accept reality and acclimate ourselves to address the cancer as best we can. Rather than ignore the elephant in the room, Marcia had a more direct approach. She preferred to walk straight through the storm with eyes wide open. Just as she advised major clients in crisis, she wanted to know things as they were, without slogan or spin.

Given the dire circumstances, we wanted to avoid running through a path of well-meaning cheerleaders, both medical and personal, telling us, "You can beat this," only to find a cliff on the other side. We wanted to map out the possible terrain ahead, whatever it might be. We wanted to know how things might play out, whether or not treatments worked, whether Marcia would survive three months, three years, or longer. We wanted to get prepared so that we could experience her remaining time as we saw fit, not in accordance with a perspective projected upon us by others, however well-intentioned their desires were to lift our spirits.

We did not buy into the "gotta have a good attitude" mantra. We found it artificial and simplistic. We did have a good attitude, but it was based on a deep reverence of the value of

Marcia's life, not a mechanical act of fighting and ignoring ominous data.

And we did fight. We did more than fight. We left no stone unturned. Marcia withstood the most blistering chemos. Under the supervision of her oncologist, I gave her subcutaneous injections of investigational medication in the morning and in the evening. She had an invasive liver biopsy to test out how new therapies might perform against the extracted tumor cells. We had Marcia's oncologist work out dosages with a knowledgeable pharmacist of the human form of an antiparasitic compound used for dogs. Marcia took various natural remedies that were supported by favorable data, as advised by integrative medicine specialists.

We covered the field on the medical front and even ventured into uncharted waters. We did so thoughtfully and always with the periscope up to see above the horizon and get ready should treatments fail. The problem is that the medical options are scant and inadequate.

Marcia and I understood the issues many have with the "fight" metaphors, but we were OK with the concept of fighting cancer as a medical malady. The issue we had is that life is bigger than a medical disorder, and even if cancer takes down a patient, the patient still wins. A win is not necessarily defeating the cancer. A win is having lived a good life, one to be proud of at any level.

So we sought to rise above the illness, at least in our thinking. A stage 4 pancreatic cancer diagnosis leaves precious little time and opportunity. So, within its limits, we felt we had no choice but to distill the wonders of life, identify our core values, and live them out. Whatever else was going on, this was the moment of truth, when the meaning of our time on earth brightens in intensity. For Marcia, that meant crystallizing how she wanted to experience her remaining days and what she wanted to pass on. With her diagnosis, the dress rehearsals, what-ifs, and reflexive aphorisms that script our usual behavior were over. Given the absolute nature of impending finality, we discovered who we actually were and exactly what composed our fundamental values. Now was the time to act on those values and let perception and small stuff go.

It made no sense to us to complain about our lot. *Of course* we wondered why this was happening, especially to someone as good as Marcia. *Of course* there were moments when we felt like we got stuck with the short straw. All sorts of emotions flooded our thoughts, especially during the otherworldly first days. While we regularly broke down and felt lost, we had no choice but to adapt to the realities of our circumstances and make the most of it.

As we read more, spoke with more experts, and became more knowledgeable, we understood we were not alone. Pancreatic cancer happens. We learned that many people spanning a broad age range had succumbed to it—public figures like Supreme Court Justice Ruth Bader Ginsburg (eighty-seven), Aretha Franklin (seventy-six), John Hurt (seventy-seven), Steve Jobs (fifty-six), Michael Landon (fifty-four), Congressman John Lewis (eighty), Marcello Mastroianni (seventy-two), Luciano Pavarotti (seventy-one), Sally Ride (sixty-one), Donna Reed (sixty-four), Patrick Swayze (fifty-seven), Alex Trebek (eighty), and Gene Upshaw (sixty-three), along with countless others around the globe.

We knew that the statistics were bad—median life expectancy is reported to be between three and six months—but there were exceptions, and everyone's experience is unique. We understood there were some incremental, positive developments in the way pancreatic cancer is treated, and negative statistics do not automatically apply to any one patient. As our oncologist said, "The only statistic that matters is yours." Yet the data reflecting poor longevity, heavily qualified treatment results, and limited therapeutic options were not imaginary. We would have to accept uncertainty and cherish every moment.

So we developed a plan based on Marcia's values and wishes. She believed that although at sixty-seven she was too young to die, she had already lived a rich and full life. She had a thrilling career at Rubenstein; a close, loving family; and a wide circle of friends and fans. We had taken wonderful trips to Africa, Alaska, and Iceland to witness their raw, unflinching beauty. We traveled often and broadly throughout Europe and the United States, dazzled and humbled by all we had encountered. And we had just returned from an unforgettable trip to the Middle East. Seasoning all this was the personal fulfillment we derived from impactful, nonprofit activities to help other people. Marcia would say to me, our family, and others with whom she felt close: "We're all going to die. I'm just going sooner than I expected, but I have a lot to be thankful for."

Marcia understood that she was a good person—humble, sincere, and oriented toward others—and that people knew it. She was as unaffected as it gets. Her favorite flower was an orchid, maybe because it was simple, beautiful, and stiff-stemmed. Orchids reflected her personality—low maintenance and, by appearance, somewhat of a contradiction in being erect and strong but open and exposed.

While life and death became an ongoing conversation, Marcia knew we were in this together and we were going to make the best of our fate. We could be miserable and wallow in sorrow, or we could be thankful for what we had and live out each day as best we could. We decided to be thankful and play the hand we had been dealt.

There would be challenges ahead, but we decided not to let them tarnish the significance of her life. We would not live helter-skelter, in hair-on-fire mode, panicking about every test result or disappointing development. There would be clarity, order, practicality, peacefulness, humor, and love. If the chemo didn't work—and we knew the long odds—we wanted a smooth float. No drama, nothing wasted or left unsaid. We would soothe ourselves, as well as those around us, so that their concerns could be allayed, too, by our perspective. This was all part of Marcia's Smooth River philosophy.

By way of a Medical Plan, we would research and network with the best doctors we could and access specialists for second opinions and different takes. We would intelligently go forward with the heavy-duty standard-of-care chemos, brace for their side effects, and prepare ourselves for test results to determine if they were working while consulting with our doctors and others about contingency plans if they weren't.

By way of a Life Plan, Marcia's priority was the well-being of our immediate family. We would bring our sons, daughter-in-law, and grandson closer to us and spend priceless time together. We would coalesce and coexist, without goals or judgments. We would just be present and experience one another.

Sometimes, we sat in our backyard or den and watched our adored toddler grandson at play. Sometimes, we got lost in a movie while he was napping. Sometimes, we would go to a playground or take our grandson to a nature preserve where there were farm animals he knew only from picture books. We would often go to the neighborhood schoolyard. Once we brought a basketball and wouldn't leave until Marcia hit a shot. It took only three tries. If Marcia wanted to speak about her cancer or prognosis, she did. Much of the time, she just wanted a sense of normalcy and to put the cancer in the background.

Given the life-threatening nature of the illness and the intensity of the frontline chemo to come, Marcia informed her firm that she had to take a medical leave of absence. Not being able to handle client matters in the regular course but wanting to stay informed and distract herself from chemo's virulent effects, she spoke with her colleagues with some frequency. A multidimensional, decades-long career and the concomitant connections with hundreds of clients and coworkers do not just come to a full stop. So many people were distraught by the news of Marcia's illness. In many ways, she was a light, a source of humor, and a font of good judgment that brightened the days of many of her colleagues. They and Marcia needed to continue their interaction, albeit on a more limited basis.

Marcia had a special relationship with Howard Rubenstein. Both he and his son Steven, who had taken over the firm's helm, stayed in close contact and made her know how important she was to that organization and its success. They had given Marcia a life, a very full one. I was married to her, but I knew that I shared her with the Rubenstein firm.

We also communicated with family and friends in a candid but sensitive manner. We understood that while we had to adapt, others would have a hard time absorbing our news and could have a more harrowing view of it than the more balanced Smooth River one we had arrived at. We knew how foreign our perspective would sound, so we intended to soothe people and let them know we were OK so they could be too. We also wanted to set the tone for how we wanted to be treated and the cancer viewed. This was how we informed friends early on (Day 9):

FROM: Richard S. Cohen
SENT: Thursday, September 12, 2019 7:36 PM
SUBJECT: Marcia

Dear Friends,

There is no easy way to say this. Last week we got devastating news. Marcia has stage 4 pancreatic cancer, meaning it spread and is inoperable. It was likely incubating for months asymptomatically.

The first 48 hours were surreal, of course, but last Friday we regained some balance after experiencing great medical care and adjusting to the new reality (a work in process). After lots of tests, yesterday we met for the first time our pancreatic cancer team and developed the medical/chemo plan, which starts next week.

We are working on the life plan and this involves trying to experience a sense of normalcy (and humor), filling days with purpose and setting reasonable short and midterm goals. Marcia spent over 41 years at Rubenstein, trained scores of people and developed a large circle of admirers. This is just to say, with a great career and great family and friends, she is coming to terms with mortality using the same rational, clear-headed frame of mind that is her DNA. And who knows what the future holds?

We are going forward a day at a time. It is comforting to have you as friends.

Warmly,
Richard

Until Marcia's body and mind gained some form of stability with the chemo, she couldn't have much company because of pain, nausea, discomfort, and the personal space needed to safely steer through the rapids of turmoil inside and around her. She understood she had earned the goodwill of extended family and friends and knew they would understand if she conducted this period her way.

She was so comfortable in her skin that she could be just who she was. During her precancer life, she was entirely at ease being the first to leave a party or guiding a group conversation back on track when someone monopolized it. Like her father, it was no big deal for her to ask for ketchup at a high-end restaurant to make steak or chicken taste better. Offending the chef or not being a foodie didn't enter her mind.

For three years, she had salmon nearly every night and didn't worry what others thought about it.

She had nothing to prove, no one to impress, no image to live up to. She just wanted to play things out as she saw them. After a few weeks, when we got our footing, some close friends and family visited. In a gentle way, I prepared them ahead of time that Marcia would tire easily, would not be up for a formal meal, might at any time be hit by sharp pain that would require her to seek privacy, and that unless she wanted to discuss her situation, conversation that worked best centered on everyday, ordinary topics—not cancer. It could get wearing for Marcia to have to repeat the ins and outs of her situation too many times. Otherwise, I kept people apprised of key events by email and phone. These communications were fanned out to others who were interested.

Neither of us reached out from a sense of obligation or expectation that people might have as to how we should conduct ourselves. Rather, our motivations were friendliness, compassion, and love. We felt those surrounding us would feel bad for us and be wounded themselves in some way by Marcia's illness. Understandably, many would be at a loss for words and not know how to express themselves. We wanted to tend to them but also make clear, as best we could, that we were going to rise above the cancer and didn't want to be pitied or looked down on. A few times, we heard some folks say things like: "It must be so terrible," or "You must be going through hell," reflecting their sense that we were emotional basket cases or projecting what their reaction might be under similar circumstances. We didn't want to be dragged into a misery others might, quite naturally, conjure up and impute to us. To some, we sought to explain our Smooth River mindset, but we didn't stress out over any need to convince anyone of anything. We were comfortable that we were in our own zone, no matter what others thought.

During the first two months after Marcia's diagnosis, I worked most mornings in my office in nearby Tarrytown, New York. But then my mind centered on Marcia. I began to think of her alone, and I wanted to be with her. I would often ask her what she wanted for lunch and pick up food on the way home. Eating was such a hit-or-miss proposition—the cancer and the chemo not only messes up your entire digestive system, it can wipe out your sense of taste.

Even when I got home, Marcia opted to be by herself. Taking a break from cancer world, she might watch a movie, read a book, or speak by phone with family, friends, and colleagues. It was comforting for each of us to know that the other was close. Over time, except for errands I had to run, I stayed in the house all day, but always gave her space.

As part of our short-term Life Plan, we tried to get out every afternoon to take a scenic walk or drive. Given Marcia's love of waterside settings, we strolled along the Hudson River, Long Island Sound, and the Bronx River. Some days, we walked laps around the high school track to strengthen her muscle tone, enhance her metabolism, and aid her digestive problems. (Walking gets your stomach muscles moving.) A few times, a personal trainer came over to help with special exercises and nutrition.

Every night that Marcia was up to eating some dinner, we ate by candlelight and listened to music. It didn't matter that many days we ate before 6:00 p.m. Marcia conked out early. It wasn't until October 11 (Day 38) that she felt well enough to suggest we go out for dinner, our first time in a restaurant since the diagnosis. Taking advantage of opportunities as they arose, if Marcia had a window of relief from pain and nausea, we hopped in the car to do something. If the moment struck at 4:30 p.m., that was when we had a light, early dinner. We liked being alone in a quiet restaurant. Dinner was not drawn out. It took less than forty-five minutes, and we often left with Marcia taking home a doggie bag full of food. The amount she ate and the time we spent at the table weren't the point. It was the experience of consciously enjoying the food, everything that came to our senses, everything about everything. It was about getting out and appreciating all the details we used to take for granted and maybe didn't notice. That was a Smooth River experience.

For medium-term goals, because we were not able to predict Marcia's physical capabilities, comfort level, or longevity, we could only plan a few weeks out. More than a year before the diagnosis, we had bought a fixer-upper waterfront home near Clearwater, Florida, where we had planned to spend more time as we got older. This was to be our dream getaway to share with our sons and their families. The house was a labor of love; for months prior to the diagnosis, Marcia and I had poured ourselves into finalizing a design that was clean, unpretentious, and functional—i.e., like her. The house was in the final stages of renovation, and our close-knit team of contractors pulled out the stops to finish up so that Marcia and I could sleep in it for the first time. We scheduled Florida trips between chemo sessions and made arrangements with a Clearwater hospital should an emergency develop while we were there. We wanted to see the house completed, binge-watch dolphins and pelicans, walk while holding hands on nearby Indian Rocks Beach, eat early dinners at intimate restaurants, luxuriate in painted sunsets, and escape into adventure movies. We wanted to share experiences that had always been part of our lives and remind ourselves of who we were. We wanted to partake in the wider world, the world beyond cancer.

We would develop a number of projects designed to fill Marcia's remaining time with purpose. A passion of ours was helping disadvantaged minorities and creating bonds with people from other cultures. Helping others was a core tributary of our Smooth River. It broadened our outlook beyond the illness and imbued us with the feeling of doing good.

Another tributary was her sense of humor, which Marcia kept to the end. She was so quick-witted and enchanting, she made doctors and other medical personnel smile when they attended to her. Many stopped in just to say hi. One time, when several doctors flanked her stretcher as she was being wheeled into the operating room for an endoscopic biopsy, she quipped: "I didn't realize I would be surrounded by so many doctors here. It's a good thing I wore makeup." To a friend who was undergoing chemo and wanted to visit near the end, Marcia said: "You can come anytime. I'm so tired of speaking to people who don't have cancer." And when we were at home and she was too weak to take a walk, she said: "No matter what, I always have strength to throw stuff out at the village dump." She lived clean.

Believing that Marcia's life would be short-lived, we saw every day as precious. Our Medical Plan was a core guide for living out the time ahead of us. But the larger Life Plan that took into account all the intangibles that fill our time on earth enveloped it. For us, the sweeping approach we formed to deal with stage 4 pancreatic cancer—the Smooth River—was so much more enriching and courageous than a routine track that avoids subjects many deem too uncomfortable and defeatist to talk about. For us, the Smooth River embraced the fight against cancer as part of a wider expanse.

However it may be applied by others, whatever their means or circumstances, the Smooth River makes the space and cleans the windshield to consider every factor involved with serious problems, be they medical or otherwise. It gave us comfort and strength, bathed us and purified us. Marcia and I would stay within its gentle waters to the end. I remain in them.

4. Getting the Diagnosis

To everything there is a season, and a time
for every purpose under heaven.
~Ecclesiastes 3:1

A few days after returning from our Middle East adventure, Marcia felt some stomach pain but couldn't identify its exact nature. After the pain persisted for a week, she reached out to her gastroenterologist to let him know about some unusual bloating and gas she was experiencing. It was not without some trepidation. Marcia shared Woody Allen's phobia about cancer. He once said in the movie *Deconstructing Harry*, "The most beautiful words in the English language are not 'I love you' but 'It's benign.'" With some humor but also concern, Marcia asked her GI if her stomach pain was cancer.

Her GI suggested she see a nutritionist and get a breath test for small intestine bacteria overgrowth (SIBO), a condition whereby bacteria that normally grow in other parts of the gut start growing in the small intestine. In an email on July 30 (more than thirty days before her diagnosis), he wrote it was "not cancer!! Gas is usually diet related." The SIBO breath test came back positive, and Marcia was prescribed antibiotics, the standard SIBO treatment. But after the antibiotics failed to alleviate her stomach issues, Marcia was called in to take a blood test a few days before Labor Day.

That Saturday (August 31), while Marcia was in Litchfield, Connecticut, for the long weekend with our son, daughter-in-law, her mother, and our thirteen-month-old grandson, her GI called her to say there were some questionable aspects of her blood test results and Marcia should take a CT scan the day after Labor Day—meaning in three days, meaning as soon as possible. Not jumping to conclusions but having bad premonitions, Marcia took the scan that Tuesday morning (September 3). Shortly after she left the diagnostic imaging center, she got an ominous call from her GI. He wanted to meet with her later that afternoon. Sensing something was wrong, terribly wrong, I came down to Manhattan and met Marcia for coffee, our heads spinning with dread. The two-block walk to the doctor's office was like a zombie march. While we were not sure of the test results, we knew we were being asked to take the steps when really bad medical news was about to be delivered.

We met in a small office, and before any words were spoken, the GI's body language and lack of eye contact said it all. Right there, the news you never want to hear filled the air like pesticide vapor. Things had been going so well in our lives. Both Marcia and I had proven ourselves professionally and cultivated wide circles of business, personal, and intercultural relationships; our new house in Florida was almost ready; and most importantly, we had a wonderful family. We were looking forward to new, productive phases in our lives. Now all of that promise was shattered.

The CT scan showed pancreatic cancer that had spread into her liver and stomach lining. There was a large, cystic mass identified in the body/tail of the pancreas measuring 3.5 centimeters by 3.9 centimeters by 4 centimeters and multiple masses identified within the liver and the mesentery (a membrane that attaches the intestine to the abdominal wall). The pancreas is only about six inches long. About one-third of it was now home to a deadly, aggressive tumor.

The pancreas and its function can seem relatively esoteric, at least to laymen. A small, flattish, pear-shaped gland, it is tucked away deep in the abdomen where it is overshadowed by more prominent neighbors. The pancreas lies hidden behind the stomach, and, almost like an afterthought, it is squeezed in near the small intestine, liver, spleen, and gallbladder. Even its function is collateral, being more of an enabling organ that assists in the processes of others. It's like a gas pump, providing essentials required for the body to operate; it is needed for life.

The pancreas's "supporting actor" function is to secrete enzymes and hormones. The enzymes are juices crucial to digesting food. The pancreas releases them via ducts leading to the upper part of the small intestine, called the duodenum. The hormones that the pancreas secretes flow into the bloodstream, and there they regulate blood sugar levels and stimulate stomach acids. Without the proper functioning of the pancreas, the body would starve for essential nutrients, and insulin would not be produced in sufficient quantities to balance glucose levels, resulting in diabetes.

Because Marcia's cancer had metastasized to other organs, it was classified as stage 4, making her ineligible for a Whipple procedure or other surgery that might extend her life for a few years or more. The Whipple procedure removes the head of the pancreas, the duodenum, the gallbladder, and the bile duct and then reconstructs a large part of the gastrointestinal tract, allowing a patient to digest food. Only if a tumor is in the head of the pancreas, has not spread to other areas of the body, and can be removed surgically will the Whipple be considered. Unfortunately, Marcia's pancreatic tumor was in the body and the tail.

The GI tried to put the news into a less-than-dismal context, saying Marcia's pancreatic cancer might not be the lethal one we had heard about. There are more benign types. But upon our researching the odds of this, we discovered that over 95 percent of pancreatic cancers are exocrine tumors (deriving from the enzyme-producing glands and bile ducts).[9] Of these, 90 percent are classified as adenocarcinoma, the most aggressive type having the worst prognosis.[10] The possibility that Marcia's cancer would be of a less dangerous type was remote.

We drove home stunned and adrift. Our world, which we had spent decades building, had just been crushed into broken elements we had little control over. Going forward,

---

9 "Knowledge, Understanding and Awareness of Pancreatic Cancer," SEENA Magowitz Foundation, https://www.seenamagowitzfoundation.org/pancreatic-cancer/.
10 "Pancreatic Cancer Types," Johns Hopkins Medicine, https://www.hopkinsmedicine .org/health/conditions-and-diseases/pancreatic-cancer/pancreatic-cancer-types.

everything would be different. Everything. While my heart was beating fast and my mind was racing, I gripped the steering wheel with my hands in the ten and two position, reaching back fifty years to driver's education to find some familiar structure. Somehow, I had to rise above my mental spirals and tend to Marcia, who must have been completely lost in King Lear delirium. Intuitively, we both seemed in lockstep, each of us trying to process things on our own, make sense of the devastating diagnosis, and come together to try to create some order. We both converged on taking baby steps: getting out of our car, putting one foot in front of the other to walk into our house, climbing the steps to our bedroom, changing our clothes, and collapsing on our bed to ponder things and talk. We tried not to get stuck, finding one stepping-stone of movement and then the next.

We had a quiet dinner at home that night, but we were just going through the motions. It was as if we had to remember how to walk, how to talk, how to breathe, how to think. We had emotional vertigo and just wanted things to be the way they had been before the diagnosis.

The next few days, before we saw any cancer experts, were very lonely and surreal. The news was especially hard to take because Marcia was the essence of goodness—so accomplished, so kind, so loving, so unpretentious. I kept staring at her. How can such destruction live within a person so beautiful inside and out? I tried to hold in my tears because I didn't want to worry her, but it was impossible to either keep from crying or worry her more than she already was. Wherever my mind drifted, I had to constantly remember to put myself in her skin and experience the shock through her eyes. I wanted to provide an upbeat tenor, a strength she could lean on, but validate whatever she was feeling and the strange new world we had just entered.

The next medical step was to undergo an endoscopic ultrasound biopsy (EUS) to confirm the molecular chemistry of the tumors and to extract genetic samples to determine, among other things, whether a new, personalized medicine approach could be applicable in the future. It would confirm whether Marcia had BRCA1 or BRCA2 gene mutations, in which case a new class of targeted drugs called PARP (poly ADP-ribose polymerase) inhibitors might be able to delay the cancer's progression. Marcia was previously tested for BRCA as part of breast cancer screening and was reasonably sure she did not have the mutation and therefore was ineligible for PARP therapy.

During the EUS procedure, which was done with anesthesia, an endoscope was introduced through Marcia's mouth and advanced into her stomach and duodenum so that biopsy specimens could be taken with ultrasound guidance. The pathology results would be available within a day or so and were a prerequisite for the first visit with our new oncologist. The genetic results, however, would not be available for weeks.

The pathology lab confirmed the existence of metastatic exocrine cancer and invasive adenocarcinoma, the worst (and most prevalent) kind of pancreatic cancer.

As an ominous indicator of trouble and pain ahead, the CT scan revealed "focal thickening and induration in the lesser curvature of the stomach, suggestive of compression by the adjacent pancreatic mass." This meant the pancreatic tumor was pressing against Marcia's stomach, which would later become the source of intense pain and internal bleeding during her final weeks.

A word on diagnosing pancreatic cancer: as mentioned, there are currently no standard screening tools to identify it early. Researchers across the world are working hard to develop detection methods, but devising reliable tests has been excruciatingly elusive. Even so, stomach pain seems to be a common enough sign in certain patients and age groups to signal possible trouble, however remote that possibility may be.

Doctors are taught to follow Bayes' theorem in their assessment of the likelihood of a given disease being present in a given individual. That is, based on the knowledge of diseases that occur in certain populations and at certain stages of life, what is the probability of that disease being present in this individual, and how does that fit with the symptoms he or she is reporting? Doctors are taught that common things occur commonly, and if you hear hoofbeats in Central Park, think horses, not zebras. Yet pancreatic cancer is more common in certain types of patients than are zebras cantering in New York. While the diagnostic permutations in medicine are innumerable, it would seem that the severity of a given disease—in addition to specifics about the patient—should be part of the decision-making equation and heighten the sensitivity that a problem may exist and merit some attentive thought.

Doctors are often reluctant to alarm patients by suggesting the possibility of serious disease to them until they have at least tried to treat the symptoms with simple remedies. But because pancreatic cancer is so deadly, it would seem to warrant early consideration in the diagnostic algorithm for evaluation of stomach pain, especially in older patients, even while more common causes are being pursued. Maybe obtaining a CT scan sooner rather than later may be an important measure to take in seeing if cancer is or is not present.

None of this is to say that an earlier CT scan would have made a difference in Marcia's outcome. It is to say, however, that just because we don't yet have a test to diagnose pancreatic cancer and just because it cannot be detected with routine maneuvers like palpation for a breast lump or prostate nodules, we should still give attention to its possible presence. Maybe there are some patterns of stomach pain that signal pancreatic cancer potential, especially among patients over a certain age, that could be studied or acted on. With stomach pain being a symptom and pancreatic cancer being a possibility—low in likelihood but high in severity—there may be some learning or judgments that can be advanced. Even if this appears like grasping at straws, we must keep trying to develop better tests and treatments for pancreatic cancer—in fact, all cancers and other disease. Until that happens, we should keep our minds open and antennae up for early warning signs.

Technically, the full dimension of Marcia's diagnosis was not delivered until the first oncology appointment—a few days after the September 3 GI visit—when our new doctor would assess the CT scan, the EUS, the biopsy results, and other factors. Yet, for all the qualifications and conventional aphorisms, the die certainly seemed cast after we left the GI's office. It was as if we had just fallen through an *Alice in Wonderland* rabbit hole, one leading to an alternate universe. But this was not one of fairy-tale delight. This was one filled with terror that needed to be tamed.

5. Taking the Hit:
Adapting to the New Realities

**When we are no longer able to change a situation,
we are challenged to change ourselves.**
~Viktor Frankl

It is hard to describe the new world we entered. The challenge is not so much to portray our immense disappointment and the deep wounds it opened. Our new world certainly involved a shocking punch that knocked the wind out of us. It took a few days to realize that this was really happening and we couldn't shake our heads and make it go away. We just had to take the blow, get to our knees, get to our feet, and somehow start moving forward.

The difficulty was in explaining how we adjusted, our transformation to living on the edge without sounding glib, rehearsed, or in denial. In this cancer world, we had to acclimate to new confines and learn a new way of thinking. Coming face-to-face with the end, we came to realize that this is just the way life is . . . it's not endless. We never had to think about it before. But now we did and, by doing so, realized that we would somehow be OK, no matter what.

A few days after hearing the crushing news on September 3, we gained some balance as we circulated through the cancer care maze. It gave us comfort to speak to oncology professionals and a handful of stage 4 pancreatic cancer patients. Marcia spoke with a few whose chemotherapy was working to stem tumor growth. One was *Jeopardy!* host Alex Trebek, who had been diagnosed not six months earlier (and who has since succumbed). Another was a woman who was playing in a weekly tennis game a year after her stage 4 discovery. Several patients were doing quite well. Yet even though there were some exceptional cases to inspire us, and incremental progress was being made in treating stage 4 pancreatic cancer, the prognosis was bleak.

After seeing a few doctors, speaking to other experts, and doing extensive research, our approach began to take shape. We were going to fight the cancer medically as long as there was a reasonable possibility of a treatment working and providing a quality of life as Marcia defined it. But no matter what we did medically, we still had to determine how we were going to conduct ourselves in, around, and through the dangers the disease and its treatment posed.

As we viewed it, we could deny reality, downplay all the implications, and push the prospects of dying from our thoughts. We could exhaust ourselves with a singular focus on "beating this thing," blocking ourselves from understanding that pancreatic cancer could very well take Marcia's life. Or we could find another way. We could take this whole crazy thing in, do the best we could therapeutically, and infuse every aspect of our being with goodness, making peace within the boundaries of what was reasonably possible.

The first course is narrow in focus and susceptible to being driven by the attitudes and platitudes of others. It puts you in the vulnerable state of letting your experience be controlled by cultural responses programmed into us, insufficiently aware of an end that may be looming. The second course, the one we chose, is expansive, self-defined, and wide-eyed. Yes, we were exposed and on our own, but we took control of how we thought, planned, and acted. Even in the face of death, we found that the smoother, more open course can lead to intense beauty and instill spiritual joy in everyday events that beforehand we underappreciated.

To us, there was just too much at stake to go off orbit and surrender to bedlam and fear. The pressure we faced revealed a different emotion in us. We became deeply thankful for everything we had, even though we continuously found ourselves on new and precarious footing. Somehow, our choice that we were going to manage this our way—along a Smooth River—stabilized us and became our safe harbor no matter what befell us.

Within our cancer world, we began to see every day as bringing about new possibilities. There were many medical appointments, but there was plenty of downtime during which Marcia read books, especially those dealing with dying and the meaning of life; watched movies and Netflix series; FaceTimed with family, friends, and colleagues; and took field trips with me. We had heartrending conversations that were forthright, open-ended, and tearful. Often, we were temporarily drawn into an abyss of bewilderment and self-pity, without answers. This was just too hard to believe. But after a while, we realized that we could let it all hang out, allow the tears to flow, and visit the recesses of unimaginable sorrow. We didn't wail. We just wept and stared at each other, knowing that we were surrounded by forces that offered no guaranteed escape but understanding that deep beneath the surface there was a calm place to put things in perspective. Like diving into water, after submerging for a while, you surface again. We came to understand that the ups and downs on the emotional graph were part of the process, a rhythm that was training us to see our situation with more complexity and maturity, as well as to expand our tolerance levels and our strength to take on what was before us.

As we adapted to cancer world, we took pains in how we communicated with others. Family and friends, I'm sure, felt anguish about Marcia and me and the wound she might leave in them if the illness took her life. Seeing our lot as tragic was entirely understandable and precisely how Marcia and I would have viewed a friend who was suddenly gripped by life-threatening illness. Yet when this is happening to you, everything changes. You are thrust into a completely different sphere, with different timelines, different goals. You are pressed to reset your guideposts, your language, your view of life, and the world. It's a crash course in entropy management, with no ways of escape other than adjustment.

Feeling bad, friends, family, and colleagues wanted to embrace us. Gestures of kindness often took the form of wanting to visit, deliver food, send gifts, or run errands for us. Some of our friends wanted to form teams of people to take care of our needs. We were deeply moved by all of this, but, with our new, Smooth River perspective, we had to caringly explain that what mattered most to us was just the intangible of knowing we were in people's thoughts and prayers. It was so comforting to know we were supported.

The reality was that Marcia needed private space—her stamina was limited, and there was no way to predict when pain or nausea would erupt, so visits had to be select and short. As best we could, we wanted to retain a sense of normalcy, meaning doing things for ourselves and not becoming invalids—until circumstances dictated otherwise.

As our story spread since Marcia's death, people dealing with their own turbulent time have asked me how they might tap into a Smooth River approach. I tell them they don't have to have a crisis management background or engage in volumes of reading. Marcia certainly was no superwoman; she had vulnerabilities, self-doubt, and insecurities like everyone. We all have qualities and experiences to draw on. We already have what it takes. All we need to do is to open our mind, our heart . . . and, of course, our eyes to see what is already in front of us. It simply involves being open to a new approach, in effect trying on a corrective lens to see the world more clearly. In cataract surgery, one of the most prevalent surgical procedures in the world, a new, intraocular lens called an IOL is inserted to replace a clouded-up lens in your eye, thereby enabling clear vision.

Perhaps we should call our way of looking at things an SRL—a Smooth River Lens.

Anyone can enter the Smooth River by just unplugging, getting off life's treadmill for a few minutes, stepping outside your own shoes, and viewing your own circumstances as a thoughtful, sensible person would from the outside.

Getting swept away by the winds of crisis or stress and losing sight of the wider picture is an age-old dynamic. Of the many notable examples of this is the Old Testament story of Hagar. At Sarah's urging, Abraham banishes Hagar and Ishmael (Hagar and Abraham's son) to the desert. When the water Abraham gave Hagar ran out and she cried to God that she and Ishmael would die, God opened her eyes to see a nearby well of life-sustaining water. The passage is commonly interpreted to mean that the well was there all along but that Hagar had been too blinded by her own tears and resignation to see it. God helped Hagar see a new approach to her hardship, which enabled her to carry on.

Religious leaders, psychologists, and advisers of all kinds constantly counsel us to change how we view a problem so that we may unlock constructive ways of addressing it. The ability to adjust to new circumstances and try a different perspective in the face of challenge is part of the package we humans are born with. We just need to free ourselves from our habitual conduct and tap into the potential we already have.

Smooth River thinking can be adopted by anyone at any time under virtually any circumstances. It simply means thoughtfully assessing a situation—medical or otherwise— understanding the realities involved, making adjustments, taking constructive action within the confines of what is feasible, and preparing for all reasonable outcomes. It may mean accepting hard realities and making the best of a situation. It may mean making the best of your life, one shortened by illness.

6. Stepping into the Breach to Manage Care and Life

The best way to not feel hopeless is to get up and do something. Don't wait for good things to happen to you. If you go out and make some good things happen, you will fill the world with hope, you will fill yourself with hope.
~Barack Obama

Professionally, Marcia worked mostly on a project basis, managing crises and other extraordinary matters for clients, and I represent medical technology companies in corporate merger and acquisition transactions. Both lines of work involve servicing clients, protecting their interests, diving into new subjects, and immersing ourselves in all facets of the situation. We are always coming in as outsiders and always respectful of tradition and precedent, but always seeking ways to create solutions that are customized to the challenge at hand.

So now Marcia was the client and pancreatic cancer the situation. Marcia and I sought to learn everything we could about the cancer on the fly. We researched and read a lot of material, but what quickly became apparent was that there were many loose ends and much imprecision because of the complexities of this variety of cancer and its woefully inadequate remedies. (Not too long ago, pancreatic cancer was considered an orphan disease and off the radar in terms of institutional funding. It was only within the past twenty years with the advent of the Lustgarten Foundation that research dollars rose above squinting levels, but far more amounts and attention are needed.)

Given the dire state of affairs, even if chemo extended Marcia's life as we hoped, its pulverizing side effects required another person to manage her care, the many clinicians treating her, and the surrounding terrain. There was no issue in our case. Marcia would soon be severely impaired and facing the seam between life and death, but she would not be alone. I was there to be her partner and care coordinator. We were ready to take this on together.

Others may not be as fortunate to have a ready, willing, and able loved one or friend to step forward. But optimally, someone close to the patient needs to be an advocate and navigate health care's complicated course. Otherwise, the patient is defenseless, and his or her judgment could be compromised by the effects of the cancer and chemo, the disorientation of pain medication, and the whole ordeal.

I knew what to do in terms of networking with top doctors and researching the field. What I had to learn quickly, however, was to subordinate my own personality and not substitute my judgments for those of my wife. Several years back, Marcia had suggested we both read the relationship-improvement classic *Men Are from Mars, Women Are from Venus.* Among its understandings is the idea that men may be bottom-line oriented and women may be more about process, wanting to talk sometimes without resolution. One of the most challenging aspects of our new world was to let go of myself and to listen to her, to let her talk about whatever she wanted to, and to give her freedom to express her anxieties, fears, pains, and wishes without my seeking to fix things. Often, I can research a problem and make a quick, efficient decision because it resolves the matter and gets it off my checklist. This was a different situation. As much as I wanted to cure pancreatic cancer, or at least beat back this monster and resume our former lives, all we could do was deal with the invader that was ravaging Marcia's body within the realms of what was medically possible.

Thank God Marcia set the tone and softly lit up the route forward. She wanted to talk about everything that was happening, or might, including the likelihood of her early demise and what dying would be like. She was very clear that she did not want to be defined by tragedy. She had the confidence to know her family loved her and that she had led a full and complete life. This self-recognition gave her freedom to discuss everything.

At first, it was hard for me to just be quiet and let her talk. My own defense mechanisms operated to shield me from confronting the prospects of her dying and to move morbid conversation to more upbeat subjects. But I quickly realized that if I didn't give Marcia freedom to speak as long as she wanted about whatever she wanted, I was keeping her in a prison to grapple with these life-in-the-balance subjects by herself. I was doing exactly what I wanted to avoid—leaving her to face this by herself. And by freeing her to speak about dying and therefore living, she gave me an extraordinary gift. She taught me that letting go of my own fears about her dying and just listening to her without interruption would not only not harm me, it would liberate both of us. It freed us to talk about everything and to leave nothing unaddressed. Like so many things, what I dreaded in anticipation strengthened me in actuality. By her own actions, Marcia was teaching me how to live more compassionately and become a more open, caring person. Cutting the cord to my own inhibitions, I could now be her care manager on her terms.

It quickly became evident that while the health-care system is amazing, there are many gaps that need connecting, whether you are seeing clinicians affiliated with only one institution or many. It's not the system's responsibility to keep track of everything that impacts a patient's life or his or her care. A patient's relationship with the health-care system is collaborative, like pieces of a puzzle fitting together. It's the job of the patient or his or her advocate to provide an organized account of the patient's experience so that doctors can optimize the treatment.

Still, there are so many variables swirling around that it's not easy to keep order, and even when you can, something unexpected happens—like a medication producing a severe side effect or the patient experiencing a sudden crash in blood pressure. Cancer—its care and management—is highly unpredictable.

As an intuitive reaction to the chaos, we divided our world into a Medical Plan and a Life Plan. Devising this model stems from the basic human instinct of self-preservation. Faced with foreboding danger, we needed to create a structure to contextualize the new circumstances and our response to it. The Medical Plan and Life Plan each made room for tangibles and intangibles, items that were defined and others that were open-ended. This pliable paradigm seemed to allow for every unexpected twist. It's not that the paradigm needed to be perfect, nor was it meant to set hard-and-fast boundaries or prove a scientific equation. Yet we found that having a framework, even if only philosophical in nature, was a vital part of our penchant for coherence. A critical point in this was that Marcia and I were doing something proactive—we were the architects of the big picture that encompassed and was influenced by the expert judgments of medical and other professionals. This wasn't a do-it-yourself project; we just sought some structure.

The Medical Plan organized all of the clinical information about Marcia's cancer, from how her case was to be specifically addressed to the current state of pancreatic cancer research, development, and innovation. The Life Plan really involved everything else—essentially, how Marcia wanted to live out her remaining time, however long or short that might be.

Due to the immense amount of information to process, I found it useful to keep a log to track appointments, test results, research findings, questions, symptoms, medications, and side effects and how Marcia was faring virtually every day. This was not a stream-of-consciousness diary or a journal of poetic musings but rather a chronology and record that I could review with Marcia and the medical staff. The log recorded key medical events but also certain lifestyle entries that described Marcia's energy levels and quality of life— like having dinner out, taking walks, visiting with family and friends, and going on trips. Keeping a log started as a simple checklist but soon turned into a centralized notation system to track Marcia's progress and decline. It was meant to be practical and usable for quick, on-the-spot access to core information and events. But it soon became clear how important the log was for the doctors to have a window into Marcia's experience so that they could make medical judgments informed by her activities outside the exam room, as well as by their own records.

An unexpected benefit of the log was that it also conveyed to the medical professionals who we were and the role we wanted to play in Marcia's care. Cancer care is a partnership between the medical professionals on the one hand and the patient and his or her supporters on the other. The more precise the contributions of each, the more effective and empowering the care can be. The partnership not only has clinical repercussions, it also has psychological and motivational ones. Doctors have so much to juggle; giving them organized life notes can infuse the doctor-patient relationship with more insight and synergy, which, in turn, could spark some new ideas above and beyond the standard protocols planned for the patient. In our case, for instance, Marcia's chemo schedule was adjusted to trips we wanted to take to Florida, and we regularly used the log to fine-tune pain and other medication levels.

The log represented a way for Marcia and me to participate in and exercise some influence over her treatment and her life. What we could control—the effort—we took on resolutely. What we could not control—the results—we just had to let happen, our efforts providing some comfort and pride that we were doing all we reasonably could. When a destination is too elusive to reach, sometimes reaching it is not the objective. The journey is. And this came to pass with us.

Below are some edited excerpts from the log. A more detailed spreadsheet is included in Appendix 1. These are offered as suggestions others may use to create their own version. I usually took notes on a yellow pad or in a notebook, then scanned the notes for safekeeping and entered them into a Microsoft Word table like the one below. Sometimes using Google Docs, I dictated notes into my cell phone to play back later, to process and make sure I'd captured all the nuances.

DATE	DAYS AFTER DIAGNOSIS	EVENT
9/3/19	0	CT scan results delivered–stage 4 pancreatic cancer with metastases in liver and stomach lining
9/4/19	1	EUS–endoscopic ultrasound biopsy–to validate tumor chemistry Genetic testing to determine if BRCA genes might respond to PARP inhibitors
9/11/19	8	First pancreatic oncologist appointment, Hospital 1
9/15/19	12	Blood testing (CA 19-9 tumor markers) Chemo 1, FOLFIRINOX At Suburban Cancer Center
9/17/19	14	Take-home pump disconnect at Suburban Cancer Center (affiliated with Hospital 1)

Date	Days After Diagnosis	Event
9/26/19	23	Marcia near collapse; dangerously low blood pressure Needed urgent hydration at Suburban Cancer Center
9/27/19	24	Marcia again near collapse; dangerously low blood pressure Needed urgent hydration at Suburban Cancer Center again
10/2/19	29	Oncologist meeting at Hospital 1 Blood testing (CA 19–9 tumor markers) Chemo 2, FOLFIRINOX, at Suburban Cancer Center
10/4/19	31	Take-home pump disconnect at Suburban Cancer Center
10/6/19	33	Dangerously low blood pressure Needed hydration, unscheduled, at Suburban Cancer Center
10/8/19	35	Spoke to another prominent pancreatic oncologist about FOLFIRINOX doses in relation to size of patient
10/11/19	38	Dinner in White Plains, Greek restaurant, a welcome return to salmon, fries, and Chardonnay
10/12/19	39	Dinner in Hastings, overlooking the Hudson. Pasta with vodka sauce.
10/14/19	41	Integrative cancer care appointment in NYC, took train in Advice: walk after eating, order supplements, eat big-bang-for-the-buck foods
10/16/19	43	Chemo 3, FOLFIRINOX at Suburban Cancer Center
10/18/19	45	Disconnect and hydration
10/19/19	46	Trainer
10/22/19	49	To FL; Marcia walked throughout both LGA and Tampa airports Marcia had cereal and muffin on plane and early dinner of pasta with vodka sauce
10/23/19	50	Conversations with colleagues and friends while dolphin-watching Sunset walk on Indian Rocks Beach, dinner at Amici's

Date	Days After Diagnosis	Event
10/25/19	52	Visits with FL friends; flew to LGA
10/28/19	55	CT scan, Hospital 1, Manhattan
10/29/19	56	Spoke with patient advocate, Hospital 1

We found that each oncology appointment involved important information, be it technical or more general. We did feel some pressure to use our limited appointment time wisely, knowing oncologists have a full caseload, each case involving a multitude of factors, including hard science and soft psychology. While we didn't feel shortchanged, it pays to plan ahead and be efficient, a practice that also respects the doctor's time and engenders goodwill. We brought hard copies of our log and prepared a written list of what we wanted to discuss a day or so before a visit so that we could refine our questions before the appointment. Some of the key questions and areas of discussion we always planned for were:

- The status of the cancer
- The status of chemo and other cancer treatments currently offered and in the pipeline
- Test results, their meaning, and their timing
- Status report on Marcia's recent experiences with cancer symptoms and chemo side effects
- Effectiveness, interactions, and side effects of each medication taken
- Pros and cons of different chemos and other approaches
- New clinical trial and experimental approaches

- Different treatment outcomes, their probabilities of success, and the amount of living time each might add
- Quality-of-life issues—how Marcia's remaining time may play out under different scenarios
- Estimate of her life expectancy
- The doctor's overall thoughts and recommendations on any and all related subjects
- Scheduling the next appointment

Medication management is a world unto itself in terms of each medication's purpose, brand and generic names, dosage, time of day to take, side effects, interactions, effectiveness, and other factors. Marcia handled her own medications until the final few months when she became too debilitated and needed help. Medication management is so complicated that I've dedicated a chapter to it, "Managing Pain and Other Symptoms: The Rotation of Pill Bottles."

An important part of the work that a patient and his or her family should do is network with resources related to the patient's condition. For pancreatic cancer patients, we found several organizations to be helpful. These and other organizations are listed in Appendix 3 and the Smooth River website, www.smoothriver.org. Although we conducted our own internet research and spoke with several oncologists who were not treating Marcia, we discussed all the information we gathered with our own doctor rather than go it alone. We told our oncologist everything. We understood that much of the information we gathered was qualified and related to a particular state of affairs, which might have been different than ours. We found that our oncologist, like we assume all do, entered the field with an open mind to help patients and would like to hear their input, questions, thoughts, and yearnings, no matter the source or nature. Both the patient and the medical team benefit by getting everything on the table and encouraging an ongoing, open interaction.

But we discovered that not every oncologist is right for every patient. Given the delicate nature of terminal illness, we found that fit was vitally important in the doctor-patient relationship.

7. Choosing Your Doctor Carefully

**The good physician treats the disease;
the great physician treats the patient who has the disease.**
~Sir William Osler

Right after Marcia's diagnosis, we did our best to find an experienced pancreatic cancer doctor in the New York area. We live in Westchester County, less than an hour from Manhattan by car or commuter train. Being in such close proximity to world-class cancer experts, we wanted an oncologist who specialized in pancreatic cancer, had access to the latest research and clinical trials, and was regarded so highly by the industry and his or her peers that he or she innovated new trials as a principal investigator. We also wanted to go to an institution that was geared up for cancer care by way of having state-of-the-art chemo suites, resources, staffing, and processes.

We learned quickly that Marcia would likely need chemotherapy, and although we did not know how frequently it would be administered, the duration of each session, or the number of sessions involved, we wanted to supplement our main Manhattan-based cancer center with an affiliated facility closer to home. In that pre-pandemic time, traffic in and out of the city could slow to a bumpy crawl, made all the more frustrating by potholes and hotheaded horn-honkers. Having a local supplemental facility that we could get to fast proved to be vital—several times, Marcia felt faint during walks and collapsed from dehydration and perilously low blood pressure. In addition to such emergencies, Marcia needed regular intravenous saline hydrations and other medical check-ins, as well as lengthy chemo sessions. Although large, academic hospitals may be home to top oncologists and cutting-edge research, surgical procedures, and medical training, they can be a beehive of high-volume, frenzied activity and may not provide the most serene atmosphere to calm the patient's soul. We would do whatever we had to for Marcia's care, but it would be far more relaxed and comfortable to have a competent facility close to home for routine care . . . and exigencies.

The medical institution we initially chose, Hospital 1, is a highly regarded provider of cancer care. Because of its esteemed oncological focus and a renowned pancreatic oncologist there (Dr. A), it seemed the logical choice to direct Marcia's case. Plus Hospital 1 had a cancer care regional center in reasonable proximity to our home (the Suburban Cancer Center).

Some people had suggested other highly regarded oncologists. We were wary, though, of doctors who were primarily surgeons, as surgery is generally not available for stage 4 pancreatic patients, or oncologists who didn't specialize in pancreatic cancer. We did welcome referrals to out-of-town specialists who could advise us on a friendly basis without our feeling pressured to be treated by them. One such person, a leading pancreatic oncologist at a major university in another part of the country, turned into a key resource for us. We were able to get his perspective on crucial aspects of Marcia's care, as well as new treatments in development or being tested in clinical trials. His informed and candid views helped to reaffirm our Medical Plan and provide additional context while reminding us that different experts take different approaches and have different personalities.

Identifying an appropriate oncologist and hospital is just the start. It may be hard to get an appointment with your doctor of choice. We were lucky that our friends' son was a fellow at Hospital 1. He helped set up an appointment with Dr. A's younger associate, Dr. B. We were disappointed not to be seeing the renowned Dr. A, but we were assured that Dr. B and Hospital 1's other pancreatic oncologists met regularly and reported to Dr. A, so we thought we were buying into an entire team of experts.

Hospital 1 advised us that we couldn't schedule an initial appointment unless it first received the CT scan, as well as the results of the EUS (endoscopic ultrasound biopsy). That took a few days to process and have transmitted to Hospital 1. Marcia and I assiduously made sure that Hospital 1 got what it needed on a stat basis so we could see our oncologist as soon as possible. The appointment was scheduled for September 11 (our 9/11, Day 8). This was the pivotal meeting we had been longing for—the meeting when we expected to be embraced by an expert pancreatic specialist who understood the needs of a newly diagnosed, stage 4 pancreatic cancer patient for information, advice, understanding, and compassion.

Marcia had—and I have—pretty good people skills, having worked with clients in crisis situations for decades. And we both understood that people have only one chance to make a first impression. So we carefully followed Hospital 1's prerequisites to make the appointment and get the staff the needed test results so that we could meet the person we expected to be our partner in saving Marcia's life, or at least extending it. We both imagined breathing a sigh of relief when the doctor entered the treatment room, at last meeting our trusted professional teammate, someone who would help us navigate out of this nightmare.

To our dismay, though, it didn't play out that way. Instead, after we heard the sound of rushed footsteps and papers shuffled outside the exam room door, Dr. B whisked into the room, quickly introduced himself, sat down on a stool, draped a single sheet of limp copy paper over his knee, and started his interview, the usual pleasantries getting short shrift. To be friendly and helpful, I offered him my clipboard to lean on, but he said he was fine and proceeded to ask us the most basic questions about Marcia's case, not reflecting any knowledge of the EUS and the other tests she had taken. I mentioned that Hospital 1 wouldn't allow us to make the appointment without having supplied the EUS, the biopsy results, the CT scan, and the CT disc. All of that was delivered days ahead of the appointment now taking place, and everything, including basic information about Marcia's circumstances, should have been in the file.

We were so vulnerable and now very confused that something was off with the expert into whose hands we were putting Marcia's life. As we explained the situation from scratch and sensed his harried schedule, it became apparent that he had not studied the chart and did not appear to appreciate how critical the first oncology appointment is to a stage 4 patient grasping for information. When we asked if he could understand our obvious circumstances, he blamed us for being overly anxious and abruptly exited the room in a huff, stunning Marcia and me. He left us alone with no explanation or direction.

With heads spinning and seeking to restore order, we called in his nurse and our friends' son to explain what had just happened and asked them to gently coax the doctor off the ledge, to read the chart, and come back into the room prepared. About an hour later, Dr. B returned and apologized for not reviewing the file. Marcia and I knew how to win over challenging people, but we had no idea that would include charming our oncologist.

From then on, we were forced to manage a doctor who seemed thin-skinned. He might have felt slighted that we had come to Hospital 1 expecting to see Dr. A and not him. Or maybe, being relatively young, he lacked sufficient experience with patients, possibly being more comfortable with data and research. We had no issue seeing an associate of Dr. A, as long as he or she conferred with Dr. A, was effective medically, and displayed the empathy that terminally ill patients deserve.

The next time we saw him, Dr. B said Marcia and I seemed to be faring better. Marcia rolled her eyes and whispered to me, "He doesn't get that he's the problem, not us."

The way medical records work is that the doctor writes in the clinical science information but also has license to add subjective observations without patient input. So when we asked to see the records for our own edification, we discovered that this doctor's myopic, slanted comments were included unchallenged. The fact that he had not initially reviewed Marcia's chart and was unprepared when he met with a terminally ill patient for the first time was never recorded. But his misplaced, self-serving observation that Marcia and I were overly anxious made it in.

When Dr. B came back an hour later, we all wanted to hit the reset button. With a much more accommodating demeanor (and likely feeling a bit sheepish), he explained that there were two different, heavy-duty standards of chemo combinations to consider immediately. Wishing to turn the corner, forgive the initial misstep, and center on the quality of the medical care, Marcia and I stayed with Hospital 1 and Dr. B for nearly two months, after three two-week cycles of FOLFIRINOX, one of the standard-of-care chemos. Meanwhile, Hospital 1's Suburban Cancer Center was ideal for chemo, periodic hydrations, and emergency needs.

We really wanted to have a great relationship with our oncologist, but it was a disappointing experience. We tolerated having a doctor whom we found mechanical in his dealings with us, while at the same time we had to play up to him to encourage appropriate interaction and empathy and avoid his having another fit. When Marcia called to speak with him about extreme pain, nausea, and other side effects she was experiencing, she was routed to his nurse, who explained, "That's not the way it works around here. Patients don't speak to the doctor. You have to speak to me." On another occasion, the nurse said we were disrespecting her by wanting to talk to the doctor.

During one urgent visit to the Suburban Cancer Center when Marcia collapsed on a walk due to dehydration and dangerously low blood pressure, a nurse there took issue with the way we were being treated and advocated for us. She said that whether a doctor spoke by phone to a patient was up to the doctor, and it wasn't Hospital 1's policy to force a patient to speak only to a nurse. She contacted Dr. B in our presence, and he called us back in a few minutes, apologizing for not being available.

We had heard so many good things about Hospital 1, and we wanted to feel at home there. Doctors who choose to specialize in oncology enter a field where ongoing trust and rapport matter, where expertise must be leavened by a desire to understand a patient's needs. Marcia discovered that the relationship with her oncologist colored her entire perspective (i.e., her life). She wanted a doctor who understood *her*, not just the thing growing inside her. She wanted some emotional connection, some evidence that the oncologist and staff cared and were treating her as an *individual* with unique circumstances. She wasn't looking for touchy-feeliness. Rather, she saw that cancer care did not operate as an automatic equation whereby a doctor prescribed a treatment that corrected a problem. Real care needs to be interactive and dispensed on a customized basis with patient input by way of symptoms, side effects, quality of life, and a host of other impacts.

There are so many gears in the health-care system. There are so many patients to treat and so few experts to do so. It must be very difficult for doctors and nurses to treat each patient as a unique being and give them their due. After all, a conveyor belt of patients is constantly passing through their exam and treatment rooms. Yet one's identity and quality of life should not get blurred out in the currents of patients, attempts to improve operating efficiencies, or for any other reason.

After three cycles of FOLFIRINOX—and obtaining results showing that it had failed to stop the cancer's growth—we described our frustrations with Dr. B to certain people in the know at Hospital 1. They in turn referred us to Hospital 1's chief patient advocate, whose job is to advance the patient's views and try to resolve them. That call took place on October 29 (Day 56). We were reticent in opening up about this because of our doctor's sensitive nature, but Marcia finally decided that she would rather live a shorter life under the care of an oncologist with whom she was comfortable than an oncologist whose personal skills seemed forced and insincere. Marcia could not get over the fact that at our first meeting Dr. B had arrived unprepared and then walked out, leaving us alone in the procedure room. A stage 4 pancreatic cancer patient being abandoned by her oncologist on the first visit was a hard image to shake. She did not want to die under his care.

In the long weeks since Marcia's diagnosis, I never stopped networking but found a balance needed to be struck. On the one hand, networking can bring about useful information and relationships. On the other, you can exhaust yourself, chasing down leads that don't pan out and overwhelming yourself with unproductive interactions. We sought to be discerning. In searching for a possible new oncologist, I came across a person who knew the pancreatic cancer terrain well and, after hearing our circumstances, suggested we consider Dr. C at NewYork-Presbyterian/Weill Cornell Medical Center (NY-Presbyterian). Dr. C gave us a completely different impression, one that was far more personalized than we had experienced. At NY-Presbyterian we would have access to the same drugs and clinical trials as we did with Hospital 1, and we were careful not to burn bridges with Dr. B or Hospital 1. The move we were considering was at a pivotal time, when Marcia's blood-based cancer markers were increasing and a new CT scan reflected continued tumor growth, meaning that FOLFIRINOX was not working and it might be time for plan B, likely the other standard-of-care chemo, Gem-Abraxane.

In switching from Hospital 1 to NY-Presbyterian and a new oncologist, we still wanted to find a local facility for fluid administration and emergencies. So I hunted for a NY-Presbyterian system hospital near our home and, after a few false starts, found Lawrence Hospital, a regional facility in Bronxville, about fifteen minutes from our home. NY-Presbyterian and Lawrence became affiliated in 2014, so I thought we were all set, only to learn that we still needed to find an oncologist with privileges at Lawrence. I sought out one who specialized in pancreatic cancer and hoped to find another warm professional, one who was compatible with Dr. C and OK with her being our primary doctor. And that was just what we found—an attentive, devoted oncologist whose only interest was Marcia's well-being and a very caring oncology center at an intimate hospital with a neighborhood feel but with NY-Presbyterian professional standards. Our two new oncologists had not worked together previously—and I don't think the oncology departments had either in the manner we sought. The information technology and medical record systems of the two hospitals were certainly not fully connected. So we, in effect, served as a bridge and felt gratified that we had united two really good institutions and contributed to Marcia's care (and maybe to that of others).

This two-hospital system worked well for us. We had the best of two worlds: a leading, humanistic pancreatic oncologist at a major university hospital in Manhattan and another warmhearted pancreatic oncologist, together with a talented, tender cancer team that felt like family at a small hospital close to home. This was Marcia-like. This was Smooth River.

Throughout, we consulted by phone with other leading oncologists on a friendly basis, making sure not to take too much of their time and overstay our welcome. We discovered that for the true believers—the medical professionals who enter cancer care for the right reasons—their hearts ache along with the afflicted. They are all in the struggle to find a cure and make their patients' lives easier and more fulfilling. And as to Dr. B, I am sure his heart is in the right place. We learned later that several people also felt that Hospital 1, while generally terrific, could at times operate in an overly regimented manner. No matter the patient volumes and work pressures, there is always room for improvement and we all could benefit from learning to be more attuned to the needs of others.

A lesson, whatever one's ailment may be: a doctor's personality matters, maybe more than his or her accomplishments. We found that someone who you feel cares about you and takes those extra steps to make you feel special can make a huge difference during trying times.

8. The Medical Plan: Limited Options

**Only put off until tomorrow what you are willing
to die having left undone.**
~Pablo Picasso

For the first oncology meeting at Hospital 1—the one that blew up on us—we came prepared with a list of questions for Dr. B after doing research and networking. There were so many open-ended uncertainties, we needed some grounding to develop our own thinking and formulate our Life Plan.

We asked questions along these lines:

▸ Please describe yourself professionally and the experience you have in treating patients like Marcia. How often do you confer regularly with Dr. A, Hospital 1's leading pancreatic oncologist?
▸ Please show us the CT scan and interpret the results.
▸ What does the cancer mean?

- What is the extent of coverage in each organ, the extent of metastases, and what are the implications?
- What is the estimated rate of growth?
- What are the treatment options, the probabilities of success of each, available clinical trials and their inclusion and exclusion criteria, and other innovations being worked on?
- What are the side effects of each treatment option? How does one manage the side effects?
- What is the duration and frequency of each treatment option?
- What medications should Marcia take for pain, nausea, and other symptoms?
- What is the next line of options if the primary treatments fail?
- What is Marcia's life expectancy and the estimated progression of the disease? Please provide some transparency into the future. How, in your judgment, will Marcia's life transpire?
- What is our appointment schedule?
- What questions have we not asked, and what else should we know or would you like to tell us? (We found it helpful to finish up with an open-ended question like this. It covers the patient in case some inquiry was omitted and allows the physician to be more expansive in addressing matters not yet mentioned.)

Although I didn't think of recording our oncology appointments, it would have been a good idea to do so on a cell phone app (with the doctors' permission, of course). Given the stress we were under and the urgency of the moment, it would have been quite easy for us to miss or misinterpret what we were hearing. I did, however, ask Dr. B to send us some follow-up notes in writing and the medical record to lessen just this possibility, which he did.

I also took my own copious notes. Here is my summary of that first meeting, as well as some surrounding research:

▸ Marcia has stage 4 pancreatic cancer, and it is likely incurable. While there are some success stories, the five-year survival rate is low. Actual longevity can be much shorter.

▸ Medically, the goal is to stop the cancer's growth, shrink it, and maximize quality of life.

▸ The two frontline treatments are chemo regimens. One is a four-drug regimen called FOLFIRINOX (FOL = Leucovorin Calcium, folinic acid; F = Fluorouracil; IRIN = Irinotecan hydrochloride; and OX = Oxaliplatin); the other, a two-drug treatment called Gem-Abraxane (Gemzar plus Abraxane). The chances of either working are 20 percent to 30 percent, although some clinical trial results reflect higher percentages due to filtered inclusion and exclusion criteria and other factors that may not reflect the realities of the broader population. And no matter what data shows, each patient's experience is unique, and results will vary.

▸ Because Marcia is relatively young and otherwise in good health, there is a shot she might qualify for a clinical trial that Hospital 1 is designing to substitute a pill form of the chemo, which has been shown to have dramatically fewer side effects compared with infusion. But to qualify for this trial, a frontline chemo would first have to demonstrate success. Pancreatic cancer is so severe that success is generally measured in stopping tumor progression, not necessarily reducing its size or killing it.

▸ Immunotherapies—activating the patient's own immune system to kill cancer cells—have had some success with several cancers but not yet with pancreatic cancer. The poor results to date relate to the complex tumor microenvironment and other particulars of pancreatic cancer. Yet immunotherapies are being researched, developed, and put into clinical trials.

▸ On the personalized medicine front, there is evidence that patients whose tumors have a BRCA1, BRCA2, or a similar alteration may have a higher likelihood of responding to a class of drugs called PARP (Poly ADP-ribose polymerase) inhibitors. PARP inhibitors can fix small DNA defects—instances where a tear occurs in one of the two DNA strands—and deter more widespread problems from occurring. Marcia is being tested to see if she has the BRCA1 or 2 gene, but she said that tests she took years ago for breast cancer screening indicated she didn't have the gene, so PARP inhibitors would not be available.

▸ Marcia and I want clarity to know her prospects, whether good or bad. We wanted to hear things straight-up. We understood that traditionally pancreatic cancer was considered a death sentence but that recent developments improved the picture somewhat. Upon probing the new developments with Dr. B, it still seemed that for a large percentage of patients, the standard-of-care chemos are not successful in stopping the cancer's progression. And, unfortunately, there aren't many other effective options once the cancer reaches stage 4.

Given Marcia's status and the limited options for treatment, charting out the first steps was pretty straightforward. Both the chemotherapies were pretty muscular, but FOLFIRINOX was newer and even more robust, meaning it could be more effective but also induce more severe side effects. There have been several studies comparing FOLFIRINOX and Gem-Abraxane on a retrospective (not head-to-head prospective) basis. One study comparing real-world outcomes of 1,130 patients from a database found a crude median overall survival of 9.6 months for FOLFIRINOX and 6.1 months for Gem-Abraxane and less frequent emergency department visits and hospitalizations for FOLFIRINOX compared with Gem-Abraxane.[11]

Because FOLFIRINOX is so strong, it is given every other week (a two-week cycle) to enable the body to recover during the off week. Each session takes about four to five hours, as the drugs and some supplemental medications are given sequentially, not together. Plus, after the cancer center session, an ambulatory pump is hooked up to a central venous access port implanted in the patient's chest, and chemo continues for

---

11 Kelvin K. W. Chan et al., "Real-World Outcomes of FOLFIRINOX vs Gemcitabine and Nab-Paclitaxel in Advanced Pancreatic Cancer: A Population-Based Propensity Score-Weighted Analysis," *Cancer Medicine, Wiley Online Library,* November 13, 2019, https://onlinelibrary.wiley.com/doi/full/10.1002/cam4.2705.

another forty to forty-six hours at home. The patient carries the pump in a fanny pack. The port connection is supposed to be kept dry, so showering is difficult, and settling into a comfortable position for sleep that does not interfere with the pump can present another issue. When the ambulatory pump is empty, the patient has to return to the cancer center to have it disconnected and flushed out. Each time FOLFIRINOX is given, a tumor marker blood test is taken to assess cancer activity since the last chemo session, and after the fourth or fifth two-week cycle, a CT scan is done for a more definitive measurement of tumor size.

Gem-Abraxane is generally given once per week for three weeks, and then there is a one-week break to complete each cycle. Each chemo session lasts only one to two hours, and there is no take-home infusion. However, hair loss is a much higher probability, as seen in breast cancer patients who are often treated with similar formulations.

Both chemo regimens are extremely strong toxins designed to retard tumor progression, but they also create turmoil for healthy cells and bodily functions. Acute pain, nausea, constipation, diarrhea, fatigue, severe energy loss, and neuropathy are all side effects that can knock a patient out.

Willing to tolerate the chemo and its aftermath in the hope of achieving some success, Marcia opted for FOLFIRINOX because it seemed to demonstrate more promising results. Still, she understood that FOLFIRINOX sometimes worked in some patients and Gem-Abraxane in others, and the prospects of either succeeding were well under 50 percent (20 percent to 30 percent, as told to us).

Chemo treatment for pancreatic cancer patients may last as long as the patient can endure it or the person passes away. A small percentage of patients may obtain remission and be able to stop chemo or qualify to join the clinical trials that substitute the far less toxic chemo pill for the infusion drip. However, chemo pills are experimental, with results yet unknown.

The bottom line is that a stage 4 pancreatic cancer patient has limited options and can be locked into some form of chemo regimen for the remainder of his or her life. Unlike some cancers, where hair loss is considered temporary because there is a somewhat predictable end to the chemo and remission is a good possibility, with stage 4 pancreatic cancer, if you lose your hair, that is the way you may be until the end. Terminal illness is such an invasion of everything you hold dear, but most of all your sense of self and dignity. If Gem-Abraxane had a distinct advantage, Marcia would have chosen it even if she had lost her hair; she wanted to take every reasonable step to live. But on balance and on the advice of her doctor, FOLFIRINOX seemed like the more powerful and reasonable first choice.

With the chemo regimen decided upon, our next step was going to Hospital 1's Suburban Cancer Center to get the access port implanted subcutaneously (just beneath the skin's surface). Once inserted, the port makes it easier to provide chemo and other intravenous medications and fluids, as well as to draw blood samples and give blood transfusions. For Marcia's port, we were given cards with the device's specifications to provide to any facility that needed to access the port on an emergency basis. The port became part of Marcia's body, literally and figuratively a lifeline. The medical staff at different facilities used it with such regularity that toward the end—Day 123—the Lawrence Hospital staff had trouble flushing it because it was dried out and clogged. Thankfully, one clever nurse remembered a trick she had learned years before. She injected the port with a drug called Alteplase, a thrombolytic medication used to treat certain heart attacks, pulmonary embolisms, acute ischemic strokes, and blocked central venous access devices. It worked.

Immediately before each chemo session, blood pressure, blood gas, weight, and other vital signs were measured, and blood was drawn to assess white and red cell counts and test for pancreatic tumor markers. The tumor marker test is called carbohydrate antigen (CA) 19–9, and it measures the presence of antigens released by pancreatic cancer cells. (Antigens are substances in the blood that cause the immune system to respond.) The CA 19–9 test is used to monitor the disease's progression. Unfortunately, no such early-screening mechanism is available to diagnose the presence of pancreatic cancer in the first place.

As mentioned, we continued for three rounds of FOLFIRINOX, each time seeing the CA 19–9 tumor marker results climb, not level off or diminish. We were told that the results could be unreliable and produce higher numbers after a chemo session because it activated tumor activity, which could be good or bad—though lower numbers, suggesting some cancer restraint, was the obvious goal. By the third FOLFIRINOX session on October 16 (Day 43), the CA 19–9 results had increased so much that Dr. B accelerated the timing of the next diagnostic CT scan, which is normally conducted after the fourth FOLFIRINOX session. Compared with the tumor marker blood test, a CT scan is considered a more accurate tumor growth assessment because it is a visualization and can objectively determine tumor size. The plan was to switch to Gem-Abraxane if the CT scan showed that the FOLFIRINOX wasn't working.

During this period, we reached out to other oncologists who were recommended to us. Dr. B planned to review the CT scan with us on October 29 or 30 (Day 56 or 57), the day of or the day before our next chemo session, and then together with us decide whether to switch on the spot to Gem-Abraxane. Multiple times, Marcia and I explained to Dr. B's wonderful assistant that if Dr. B reviewed with us the CT scan results too close to the next chemo date, we wouldn't have enough time to decide thoughtfully whether to switch regimens. There were just too many life-in-the-balance factors that needed to be carefully weighed: Given the drubbing Marcia's body was taking from the cancer and the chemo, would she be able to tolerate a new hard-hitting poison? What would the side effects be, given her depleted state? What would be her quality of life—and wouldn't defining quality of life require Marcia's informed input? What are the odds the new chemo would work and what does "work" mean given all the ambiguities? What is her estimated life expectancy with and without the new chemo? And what questions have we overlooked? It was as if we were expected to automatically fall in line with whatever the oncologist thought, without having the time and space to assess things and gain perspective. Concerned with being jammed in time to switch chemos, we posted this note on October 23 (Day 49) on Hospital 1's online portal, together with photos showing Marcia enjoying some off time to develop a more personalized relationship with the doctor:

Dear Dr. B,

Marcia was amazing yesterday, navigating thru LGA and Tampa airports w/o issue, eating breakfast, lunch, and vodka-sauce pasta for an early dinner. She drinks a lot of tea.

We want to make sure that after the CT scan on Monday there will be sufficient time to carefully consider and discuss the chemo options on Wednesday. She is having a respite in FL—and is proud to get to this beautiful place on the water—but next Monday will represent a major crossroads. We hope for good results but whatever they are, we need time to assess things. We assume you will be conferring with Dr. A and the team too and would appreciate learning the results on Monday to give us all time to process things. She is concerned that she has lost 17 pounds although she continues to eat. She thinks she feels the cancer growing.

Richard

On Monday, October 28 (Day 55), we drove to Hospital 1's main facility in Manhattan for the CT scan. The very next day, Dr. B called to report that the scan showed a mild progression, meaning that the FOLFIRINOX was not working. He recommended that we immediately switch to Gem-Abraxane the following day, Wednesday, October 30 (Day 57). For some reason, despite our previous communications, he didn't get that Marcia needed more time to consider the switch and all its implications rather than robotically hopping onto a new treatment track.

October 30 was a big decision day for us. In addition to meeting with Dr. B, we met with two other pancreatic oncologists in Manhattan to consider moving to one of them. At 10:00 a.m., we met with Dr. C of NY-Presbyterian (the angelic one we switched to). At noon, we met with Dr. B of Hospital 1, and then, at 2:30 p.m., we met with a third pancreatic oncologist, this one associated with yet another well-known medical center. During the visit with Dr. B, we took another CA 19–9 test per custom but deferred the new chemo session he scheduled right afterward because we needed more time to decide on the chemo strategy and because we might be switching doctors.

In the process of getting our minds around FOLFIRINOX's ineffectiveness and the possibility of switching to Gem-Abraxane, Marcia inquired about ways to inhibit hair loss. One was a "cold cap" cooling system, which is a tightly fitting, strap-on helmet filled with gel coolant intended to narrow the blood vessels under the scalp. This hopefully reduces the amount of chemo reaching the hair follicles. With less chemo in the follicles and the lower temperature decreasing hair follicle activity, hair loss may be less likely. While it initially seemed like a solution, on further investigation, it was complicated logistically. The process involved a third-party company to administer the coolant, the helmet could be uncomfortable and painful, and, worst of all, the system might not work.

To our positive surprise, the CA 19–9 test on October 30 (Day 57) showed a marked decrease in pancreatic tumor antigen, the only piece of good cancer news we received throughout Marcia's illness. Dr. C and other oncologists with whom we consulted thought it was reasonable to continue one more cycle of FOLFIRINOX, given that for the first time the CA 19–9 results had decreased, even though CA 19–9 results are notoriously unreliable. And, given the far better personal chemistry we experienced with Dr. C, we made the switch to her. Before resuming the FOLFIRINOX, Dr. C wanted to briefly pause the chemo cycle to conduct an invasive liver biopsy to obtain tumor cells for an organoid culture, whereby different drugs could be tested in a petri dish to see if any would be useful against growth of the tumor.

On November 11 (Day 69), Marcia had the fourth FOLFIRINOX treatment, this time at NY-Presbyterian. As planned, we had the chemo pump disconnected two days later at Lawrence Hospital in Bronxville. But by then, Marcia was considerably weaker and more fatigued. Sitting in a restaurant with a plate of food in front of her was now a chore.

On November 21 (Day 79), another CT scan confirmed more tumor growth, leaving us with a huge dilemma: After going with the most powerful chemo, which gutted Marcia but had failed to dent the cancer, should we switch to Gem-Abraxane, the hair-loss chemo, and bet on the hard-to-quantify possibility of extending Marcia's life with some quality? Or should she just live out the remaining time as is? Marcia had lost so much weight and was now pretty frail. The low odds of more chemo working and the slender benefits it offered even if it did work did not seem worth the pain and degradation, given Marcia's weakened condition and everything else at play. We had spent eighty days waiting for a turning point or at least some favorable sign, but neither came.

When you temporarily lose your hair due to a chemo that has a reasonable chance of beating back a cancer, that is one thing. It is quite another to lose your hair with a long-shot chemo and the prospects of survival slipping away. Marcia's beautiful hair was one of the last vestiges of her physical self-image and sense of dignity. Words cannot describe the gravity of the decision in front of her; Gem-Abraxane, while so deficient against pancreatic cancer, was really the only medical tool left. She took about forty-eight hours to decide, during which I took her to a wig shop to see what the artificial-hair experience would be like. After carefully weighing the possibility of gaining some basis to lengthen her life and consulting with her family, she decided she had it in her to climb higher and try Gem-Abraxane. That was not an easy choice. It showed what she was made of.

The next day, she asked her friends to take her back to the wig stop for a consult. Her friends and the women at the store actually made it a fun experience as Marcia tried on various looks; the shop specialized in cancer patients, and the assistants could not have been more compassionate. A few days later, Marcia had a beautiful wig that closely resembled her hair. The new chemo might weaken her and change her appearance, but she was surrounded by love and understood that it was her soul that counted, not the way she looked. Marcia had the inner strength to go on.

After all that, however, Marcia never had to wear the wig. The Gem-Abraxane didn't work. She said goodbye in her natural hair.

During our run through the medical currents, chutes and eddies, we sought to absorb every splash, bump, turn, and drop—we understood, with eyes wide open, the surging strength of the disease. Coming to terms with mortality enabled us to make decisions and cushion medical downers without feeling like every negative outcome meant hell on earth. Keeping our eyes on the stars but our feet on the ground, as President Teddy Roosevelt once said, helped abate the frenzy and smooth out the river.

Adjusting to the vicissitudes of terminal illness was not conducted in a vacuum or by hypnosis, mental self-trickery, or quick-fix thinking. Everything was framed within our Life Plan, a testament to the paramount importance of life's wholeness, its all-encompassing panorama. Seeing one's life as bigger than one's condition is the gateway, the core theme of the Life Plan, the core theme of this book.

9. The Life Plan:
Finding Silver Linings Everywhere

Whatever you want to do, do it now.
There are only so many tomorrows.
~Michael Landon

Years ago, when health wasn't an issue, Marcia and I had developed a motivational tool to keep the priorities in our lives in order. As a constructive exercise and with some humor, we imagined ourselves at life's end (way, way off in the future) and shared what we wanted to accomplish before it was over. (We jokingly even thought of ourselves lying in a coffin with the lid about to shut.) Intended to be a light self-kick in the rear, the image clarified the temporary nature of life, how we must imbue it with meaning while we can, get things done when opportunity strikes, and not put them off. It helped to elevate the consequential from the frivolous and remind us what we wanted our lives to stand for as opposed to the silly stuff that protects or advances our egos. We sought to concentrate on matters of character, especially how we interacted with others.

We both knew that life was more than doing things by ourselves to generate pleasure. Our joy would come from relationships and how we touched others. We certainly wanted to pass on love and good values to our family. But we also wanted to give back to and learn from others. As Jackie Robinson once said, "A life is not important except in the impact it has on other lives."

Little did we know that our motivational tool would be put into use so soon and under such dire circumstances. Whether the cancer treatments worked or failed, we had to figure out and activate our Life Plan, fast. We did not follow that old Hollywood trope of running willy-nilly, seeking to fast-forward decades of life into a few months, although this may work for some. Our Smooth River way was different. Our way was softer, calmer, more peaceful, and, to us, more satisfying, given where we were.

We didn't know how much time we would have left. We hoped the first chemo regimen would work, but our goal was for Marcia to live first through Thanksgiving (Day 86), then year-end (Day 119), and then her birthday, January 7 (Day 126), when she would turn sixty-eight. That was about the longest horizon we expected, although we would be elated if her future were longer, certainly through July 2020, when a new granddaughter was due.

Our Life Plan involved setting short-term goals and, after acclimating to chemo's body blows, medium-term ones. In the short run and as part of our regular routine, we went exploring nearby. We sought to change the scenery and mix things up by getting out of the house, applying our muscles and minds to activities in the outer world, and absorbing the restorative powers of nature. Our medium-term planning involved non-profit projects and bigger adventures. Between chemo sessions and while Marcia was still able, we squeezed in two trips to Florida to sleep, for the first time, in the waterfront house we had been renovating for nearly a year.

Given the havoc that the cancer and chemo were playing, we had no time to waste in making every day count. We continued to relish our quiet, candlelit time each evening when we would watch a movie, read books, or eat light meals when Marcia was able. Often, I brought a tray of food into our den, turned off the lights, and let the candlelight flicker while we escaped into a romantic comedy, an adventure, or even a murder mystery. We just unplugged and created a soothing environment, immersed in the moment, doing simple things that we had previously taken for granted, never particularly noticing how ripe they were with value.

Each day was a new adventure, punctuated by bouts of pain and nausea, but also by breaks in the storm and even rainbows at day's end. We tried to live each day as if there would be no tomorrow. We knew this exaggerated our circumstances until we neared the end and tomorrows became truly uncertain. But the approach helped us see every day as a perishable gift. In cancer world, standards are reset in a way that outsiders may not understand. Outsiders may see deriving pleasure in simple things as sad, evidence of a shrunken life with diminished boundaries. In our world, everything brimmed with promise.

Our family and close friends provided company and warmth on whatever terms Marcia wanted. The love and support were unqualified. Within this small circle, there were no goals, nothing to accomplish. There was just the joy of hanging out together. No entertaining was necessary. Marcia could just be. This was "off time."

But there was also "on time" when we pursued reasonable goals. I tried to be a gentle coach, recognizing Marcia's pain, incapacities, and anxieties, but encouraging outdoor activities, like nature walks and drives on nearby country roads or finding a new restaurant where we could sit outdoors and have herbal tea and carrot cake in the afternoon. As we did these things, I noticed how intent her eyes were on what was before her, how responsive her senses were. It was almost as if she were absorbing these experiences for the first time and registering how miraculous life is. Sometimes, Marcia resisted going out when feeling lethargic but was always thankful once we reached our destination, soaking in a river or pond or absorbing the sun streaming down or slowly sipping a drink in new surroundings.

On one level, the mind can only focus on one thing at a time, so we engaged in simple activities to take the focus off cancer and change the environment. We sought to activate within us the neurotransmitter dopamine, sometimes dubbed "the happy hormone" because of the sense of pleasure it engenders. We loved our walks along the Hudson River, along the harbor in nearby Mamaroneck, through the glorious Rockefeller Preserve, and to small hamlets in Northern Westchester. We also listened to a lot of music, Broadway show tunes, romantic classical instrumentals, jazz, and folk rock—Carole King, Fleetwood Mac, Paul Simon, Jim Croce, James Taylor, the Eagles, Bill Evans, and others—to bring us back to more comfortable times, to evoke good memories and ease.

Because Marcia loved being beside water, our walks in Tarrytown along the Hudson took us to another place. Like many dramatic parts of the country, the expanse of the river, the cliffs on the other side, the new Governor Mario M. Cuomo Bridge, and the entire panorama are breathtaking. It's not just the grandeur of the river or the geometric artwork of the cable system supporting the massive towers and sweeping shape of the bridge. It's also the mystical and charming place where the bridge makes shore in Westchester County. Tarrytown was settled by the Dutch in 1645, and in 1820, dreamily immortalized by Washington Irving in *The Legend of Sleepy Hollow*: the "small market town or rural port . . . known by the name of Tarry Town."

A partnership between the Village of Tarrytown and the nonprofit Scenic Hudson had reclaimed industrial sites and turned them into a magnificent waterside parkland and esplanade along the river, decorated with grass terraces, native wild plants and flowers, and rims of boulders designed for sitting and taking it all in . . . views of the Manhattan skyline to the south, the sunset reflecting across the three-mile width of water and over the hills to the west, and a historic lighthouse to the north.

During our walks by the Hudson, Marcia often needed to sit on benches to rest or sometimes brace for a fall. On one outing, I noticed some people sitting on large, uneven rocks by

the water's edge to gain unobstructed views of the sunset and
began to think about having a bench made in Marcia's honor
and having it installed close to the water for safer seating.
After Marcia understood that the bench was not a memorial
bringing forward her death but an opportunity to honor her
during her life while also providing for inspirational seating
for me and others, the idea melted her heart.

I broached Scenic Hudson about it, and they put me in
touch with the Village of Tarrytown administrators who
oversaw the area. I suggested a rather commonplace site for
the honor bench and proposed an inscription that would
mention Marcia but welcome everyone. The village administrators understood that she did not have long to live and
had grander plans. To my amazement, they offered a far more
picturesque location on a bluff under a tree with awe-inspiring
sight lines. They proposed to build a small, dedicated area
for honor and memorial benches, Marcia's being the first.
Recognizing Marcia while contributing to the village's plans
to beautify the area gave both of us a jolt of energy. The bench
inscription reads:

In honor of
Marcia Horowitz
Peace, inspiration, and healing for all

With Tarrytown being a fifteen-minute drive from our
home, I also arranged for two other benches by a duck pond
on the walk Marcia took every day to and from our local
train station as part of her commute. I sometimes sat on

one while she was napping at home and knew in the future it would be another sanctuary for me. The inscriptions on those benches say:

In honor of
Marcia Horowitz
To all those who love
the serenity of flowing water

In honor of
Marcia Horowitz
Public relations executive for 41 years
A sanctuary for longtime commuters

These projects and others conducted to help build bridges among disparate groups offered invaluable opportunities of engagement for Marcia, diversions that nourished her—nourished us both. They allowed her to reach inside herself to tap into something deeper than cancer and help create something enduring that would benefit others. It was important for her to immerse herself in something outside herself while she had the strength, focus, and time.

We found silver linings everywhere, simple pleasures we had never pondered over before, but now they drew us in, like having dinner in the late afternoon in any empty restaurant. Or studying landscapes in our neighborhood that we had passed hundreds of times without noticing. Or just doing something that seemed normal.

We kept waiting for some good news that the chemo was working—killing the cancer or at least stemming its growth. We were hopeful that we would experience an objective indicator of optimism. But it never came. The only positive sign was an ephemeral tease, the lower tumor marker result that a negative CT scan wiped out days later.

We had no long-term plans, as we didn't know how Marcia would feel, given the unpredictable effects of the chemo and the cancer. Our horizon could only be a few weeks into the future, considering the tenuous nature of Marcia's state. Yet we did want to be as outward as we could, always maintaining optimism that the chemo would work. We wanted to take flight and be a bit adventurous.

The first trip we planned was to Florida from October 22 to 25 (Days 49–52). We scheduled it after the third FOLFIRINOX treatment and left a good six days for Marcia to recuperate from it and get rehydrated before getting on a plane. The conscientious contractors rehabbing our fixer-upper house worked overtime to complete it. The house was as much a labor of love for them as it was for us. Working closely together for almost a year, we were joined together well beyond a professional relationship. Everyone developed an easy, conversational rapport with Marcia, and news of her illness hit them hard. It was as if they were part of the medical team, too, because they knew Marcia's being able to spend time in the house for the first time was part of her therapy.

We had a lovely trip. Delta Airlines helped out with trip logistics and special fares and cancellation policies for seriously ill patients. Marcia was able to walk through the New

York and Tampa airport terminals on her own, stopping from time to time to rest. We ate out all three nights at small, intimate restaurants; took walks on Indian Rocks Beach; and just hung out looking at the water. Our go-to lunch spot was Panera Bread because Marcia liked their hibiscus iced tea, a source of hydration. We met with all the contractors and a close circle of people with whom we became friendly. It was a wonderful respite that provided another window into how we might spend more time should Marcia's treatment work.

When we returned to New York on October 28 (Day 55), Marcia had another CT scan. This one showed more cancer progression. It was not the turning point we had hoped for.

A few weeks later, from November 16 to 19 (Days 74–77), we took off again to Florida. But this time, Marcia was considerably weaker and needed wheelchair assistance in both airports in both directions. The trip provided another breather and change of scenery. Yet now, because of the cancer's creeping encroachment, we mostly stayed at our house. We had some visitors, but Marcia would last only a few minutes with them due to pain and discomfort. Before we traveled, we had already scoped out Morton Plant Hospital in Clearwater in case Marcia needed hydration or other urgent services. And sure enough, we had to go. It was very helpful to have prepared for a possible visit beforehand, so we knew where to go and what to do. And like always, our log and medication list helped the providers in caring for her.

Although the waterside setting was beautiful and sun and water surrounded us, weeks later, Marcia felt that, given her incapacities, she didn't have the strength to travel again. When you are withered by disease, everything becomes an ordeal. So she couldn't return on Christmas week to host our older son and his family. Instead, to orient them, with Marcia's urging, I flew down by myself for two nights, which gave our younger son and Marcia some time together in New York. We learned that each of us had our own relationship with her and that it was good to respect that and enjoy time spent in different configurations.

As a family, we gathered for Thanksgiving (Day 86) and a full turkey dinner. We made a pretty good bird (with Whole Foods giving an assist) and had a loving and serene evening mixed with our grandson's exuberant chaos.

Marcia's appetite was like a roulette wheel, there being no certainty what she could eat. Many times, we made or brought something in, only to discover she couldn't eat it. She would apologize and ask me if I wouldn't mind cleaning up and eating by myself so that she could retreat upstairs or to our den to read or watch a movie.

For our younger son's birthday on December 9 (Day 97), we wanted to do something out of the ordinary. Marcia was game for bringing in a big-time steak, and that was what we did. Just as she had for her entire life, she squeezed Heinz Ketchup beside it. She ate only a few bites, but for a few brief moments, she was transported to a different time when a special meal accompanied a happy occasion. While the atmosphere was muted, we were able to celebrate spending quality time together, knowing that doing so would likely come to an end in the not-so-distant future.

Integral to the Life Plan was creating a legacy for Marcia while she was still with us so she could appreciate how she would live on through me and others and continue to make the world a better place. She was too weak and too modest to translate the many good things she had accomplished and inspired into some tangible form that her survivors could build upon. Doing something that would outlast her was a touchy subject because it might feel like I was treating her as though she were already gone. But Marcia's openness about everything, including her death and our family's well-being after she left us, freed me to create some enduring structures that we both could participate in while she was still able to do so. Why wait until she passed to develop some sustaining legacies for her? While she might not see how the legacies would flourish in the future, she could help plant the seeds and build the foundations for them now. I remember how she radiated with shyness but immense gratitude that together we could arrange for some initiatives to help others in her name.

When our Palestinian friend, Rahima, had hosted us the previous summer in Israel, Jordan, and the West Bank, we had talked with her about the possibility of setting up a small nonprofit to facilitate relationship-building among Muslims and Jews both in Israel and in the United States and otherwise help the disadvantaged. When we were in Israel, we had even scratched down some possible names for such an organization, like Engage the Other, Engaging Partnerships, and Peaceful Interactions. Nothing seemed to hit the right chord.

For years, Marcia and I had been involved in a broad spectrum of intercultural activities. Our concept of a new nonprofit was a small, agile, and personalized effort to build relationships—and replace distortion with knowledge—among people of diverse cultures and to do so on a grassroots basis. For years, we had hosted people of other faiths and backgrounds at our home for dinner and facilitated a wide diversity of friendships among unlike people. It had been a joy to witness that heavenly moment when the proverbial lightbulb gets lit, when two people of different faiths, races, or cultures genuinely connect. For years, Marcia and I had talked about some structure to bring people together and effectuate these experiences, which then might produce societal change in some small way.

With Marcia declining and so many things to do in regard to her health, we had a choice. We could confine our focus to her health alone and stay in a dark place, or we could try as best we could to make this time really count and do everything possible to let the sun shine in. I also came to understand that our efforts to steep Marcia's world with purpose and dimension would be the foundations to carry forward her gifts and give my life purpose and dimension after she was gone.

When given time to decide on something, we often take up the time allotted to make the decision. With the compression of our circumstances requiring more nimble judgments, a name was hatched in short order for our nonprofit—Marcia's Light Foundation. I knew the name sounded Marcia-centric, and, given her humility, she would have to be convinced that it would touch people's hearts, would inspire us to do good things, and would be far more authentic than a canned name in general circulation. She thought about it for a day or so and finally said it was OK. Rahima loved the name, too, and how it carried with it the opportunity to do good guided by the inspiration of a good person.

With all that was going on and the end becoming more visible, Marcia cried with appreciation that her name would be used to illuminate the humanity and decency common to all people and that her loved ones would have some footing to carry on after she was gone. To me and my family, we were not only embarking on a lasting legacy while Marcia declined, we were developing a relationship with her soul in the hereafter.

On December 20 (Day 108), Marcia and I organized a luncheon sponsored by Marcia's Light Foundation at a local mosque after their Friday afternoon Jummah services. The leaders were so kind, allowing me to address more than 150 worshippers about our experience with pancreatic cancer so that others beset by illness would not feel alone and in the shadows. We planned to bring in Kosher pastrami sandwiches along with Halal chicken biryani dishes, but we were told that no one would eat the pastrami. We brought in two platters, together with coleslaw, potato salad, and pickles, anyway. Marcia was not strong enough to attend but got a kick out of the fact that the pastrami sandwiches went so fast there weren't enough to go around. I overheard the leader of a prominent Muslim women's organization tell her colleague that she wasn't eating the sandwich correctly. She needed to dip it into the sauce. The sauce was Russian dressing. Building relationships with "the other" is always easier with the right food. Kosher pastrami is guaranteed.

The brightness of Marcia's Light would shine well beyond her passing. Many programs have since been conducted and are being planned in the United States and overseas to pay tribute to health-care professionals during the coronavirus pandemic, build bridges among people of different backgrounds, and otherwise help the disadvantaged.

Marcia and I developed bonds with other nonprofits that help underprivileged communities. One is El Centro Hispano, which provides guidance, training, and support for the Hispanic community, and another is Mentoring in Medicine, which assists African American and other minority students in seeking health-care careers. The close personal relationships we formed with the principals of each organization continued to instill purpose during Marcia's illness. El Centro Hispano even named an early-childhood program after Marcia and me.

Throughout her illness, Marcia also regularly texted and spoke with work colleagues from Rubenstein. These interactions, so kind and warm, were always a boost to her spirits. Her colleagues delighted her with a hilarious, heartwarming video tribute to her remarkable forty-five-year career that Marcia loved. It's now uploaded on the memorial website we made for her—www.marciahorowitz.net—along with many other photos and tributes.

Setting up a nonprofit, organizing honor benches, and engaging in projects and other pursuits were our ideas to invest meaning in Marcia's limited time and inspire us to carry forward her values after she left us. Other people will have their own ideas to recognize their loved ones' legacies.

Marcia and I devised our Life Plan on our own based on our own circumstances. We didn't prepare a PowerPoint presentation or anything formal. We called it a plan mostly to people with whom we communicated. To us, we were just living and creating some order while making lots of room for downtime to absorb all of cancer's degradations.

The simple equation that worked for us was to design enduring projects that our family could collaborate on during Marcia's life, demonstrate her value and our love for her while she was still alive, offer a vision of how we would carry her legacy forward, and provide ourselves with the foundations to do so. We found it rewarding to direct our efforts to helping others, thereby doing good and instilling a higher purpose in our lives—higher than cancer.

When other people undergoing medical experiences like ours have asked for specific suggestions as to what they, too, might do, I have hesitated. What resonates for each of us is personal. But I encourage them to look deeply into what is important to them and at what can be accomplished in the patient's remaining time that can last thereafter. This is the time to unleash one's imagination. Some ideas may include video tributes much like the folks at Rubenstein made for Marcia or photographs posted to a dedicated website taken by a collection of friends and family. Organizing a food, clothing, or toy distribution for the needy or a donation for community seating, a tree, or a garden are other ideas. For those interested in education, they may consider creating a small scholarship fund or achievement award, other support for students, donating books to a library, or underwriting laptops or other supplies for underprivileged children. Consulting with small nonprofits whose mission resonates with you can yield meaningful ideas and opportunities. Being more accessible and flexible than the larger national organizations, they may propose several projects in the name of your loved one. You can also honor that person as part of a charitable walk, run, bike ride, or other endeavor or set up a GoFundMe campaign. (GoFundMe donations may not be tax deductible unless they are made to a qualified nonprofit organization.) The list of practical pursuits—culture, the environment, medical research, social justice, athletics—is limited only by one's creative thinking.

For anyone wishing to form a nonprofit, it is a bit involved but tremendously exciting and rewarding. Start by identifying a purpose that is dear to you, one that you are passionate about, and addresses a societal need in a distinctive way. While the organization can be small and simple in structure, you'll need to consult with nonprofit professionals to understand the legal requirements and other factors involved.

The key to any of these good deeds is not about scale or expense, for the project can be small and intimate. The point is to conduct a long-lasting project to honor you or your loved one. Like us, you may want to identify an underserved need and a unique and practical approach to meeting it. Speak to trusted family and friends to test out your idea and brainstorm how together you can generate the energy and excitement that would make for a successful venture, remember your loved one, and serve laudable interests.

After Marcia passed, my family discovered that all of our efforts along these lines helped to steady us during the grieving process. But when she was still with us, when the candles flickered to soft background music, when we infused her final days with purpose and meaning and her mind lit up and she smiled, when we were shaping sustainable projects together, when we, in effect, crumbled and reinvented ourselves—it was absolutely magnificent.

10. Managing Pain and Other Symptoms: The Rotation of Pill Bottles

Out of clutter, find simplicity. From discord, find harmony. In the middle of difficulty, lies opportunity.
~Albert Einstein

Given the gravity of cancer, especially stage 4 pancreatic cancer, we mistakenly thought that the health-care system would know Marcia's medication status at any moment in time via hospitals' information systems and electronic medical records. The system does not, however, provide for absolute knowledge, and there are too many variables from hospital to hospital, from doctor to doctor, from shift to shift, from nurse to nurse, from portal to portal, from day to day—and so much depends on patient feedback and sensations, which change all the time. For each patient, there is just too much data and variability to expect the health-care system to know medication status in real time.

Every time a patient sees a doctor or enters a medical facility, the staff asks for a list of drugs the patient is taking.

While this can become repetitive—as it can happen several times a day—this practice double-checks the medications the patient is taking as well as monitors their side effects. For our own purposes, Marcia and I found it essential to keep rigorous track of her drugs just to stay organized and to make sure she was taking the right ones at the right times, and we had an ample supply of each. After a while, we organized them by symptom, dosage, and when they were to be taken—at a specific time of day or as needed.

We learned that our system was so efficient that when asked by the clinicians for current medications, we simply gave them our notes. Some just took cell phone pictures of them. It became a habit to bring hard copies for the medical staff to keep in their files and to input into Marcia's digital health record. Although medical staff constantly rotates, those who knew us learned to ask if we had brought our medication log. Since we were simply keeping notes and scribbling down medication names as best we could as laymen, the printed log enabled us to correct misunderstandings and our own transcription errors while serving its primary purpose to record doses, interactions, and the efficacy of each drug.

These are my collected notes on January 13, 2020 (Day 132):

- ‣ For long-acting pain relief, Fentanyl patch 25 mcg + 12 mcg patches; every 72 hours, but can switch at 48 hours if necessary
- ‣ For breakthrough pain relief, oxycodone 10 mg
- ‣ To help intestinal digestion, Sandostatin
- ‣ For orthostatic hypotension, Midodrine 3x/day

- For "up" feeling in morning, Adderall
- For sleep, Clomipramine (75 mg), but be wary of orthostatic blood pressure
- For depression and appetite, Remeron at night
- For anxiety, Ativan
- For digestion, pancreatic enzyme pills to supplement enzymes that the pancreas can no longer adequately provide for breaking down food
- For nausea, Reglan. Stopped Zofran.
- For constipation, take MiraLAX every day, a gentle laxative. Take Dulcolax, another laxative, when needed. Also tried Senokot and Colace.
- Stop all laxatives once you go, and take MOVANTIK, which is for maintenance, designed for opioid-induced constipation in adults.
- For intestinal problems and to treat stomach spasms, dicyclomine (Bentyl)

To help us manage the medications at home, we got a pillbox with three compartments for each day so that we could load up medications to be taken in the morning, at noon, and at night and then keep track of those to take as needed. To help identify the pill bottles, I bought different color labels for our Brother P-touch label machine so the name by which we referred to a drug (such as Reglan) stood out from all the details on the label. Our go-to label color, orange, enabled us to grab a drug quickly from the more than fifteen pill bottles in the rotation. We actually had far more pill bottles, but I separated them into two large camping zipper bags for those medications we were currently using and those we might have tried but didn't work or we otherwise didn't use anymore.

Stage 4 pancreatic cancer is aggressive by its nature. The frontline chemos are so intense that they cause equally intense side effects that make it tough to tell whether pain, nausea, constipation, diarrhea, indigestion, fatigue, and other symptoms are caused by the cancer or by the chemo. Pain medications like OxyContin, morphine, Dilaudid, and Fentanyl induce nausea and vomiting. That often makes eating very difficult, wiping out one's appetite on top of one's sense of taste being smothered by the torrent of other elements roiling through the body. The mix of all these substances creates a vicious cycle: pain and nausea need to be treated, but pain medication adds to the nausea and constipation already created by the tumors and chemo. The nausea and constipation impeded Marcia from eating and caused her to throw up. Her declining appetite led to significant weight loss, and the combination of an empty stomach, reduced body mass, resulting fatigue, and bloating led to more pain. You need to eat to stay alive. But cancer, chemo, pain medication, and their side effects make it hard to do so. Not eating and its cascading effects cause more pain and nausea.

There are so many other symptoms vying for attention. Doctors can prescribe different medications to address each one, but many don't work, and they have side effects and inter-actions with others. It's very much a trial-and-error process. You try something. It may or may not help. If it does, the relief may be temporary until something else happens, causing it to be less effective or induce some other issue. For instance,

Marcia took Clomipramine, an antidepressant to help her sleep and moderate her mood, but a side effect was that it lowered her blood pressure. The dosage was reduced, and Marcia was prescribed Midodrine to address orthostatic hypotension (low blood pressure when standing). That interaction needed to be carefully watched.

Palliative care, the medical specialty dealing with pain and symptom management, is a relatively new area that is becoming more mainstream. It focuses on relieving symptoms, suffering, and stress and improving the quality of life of a seriously ill patient. A palliative care team typically includes a physician, nurse, and social worker, and, depending upon the patient's needs, a psychologist or psychiatrist, a physical or occupational therapist, a dietitian, a chaplain, and others. These specially trained professionals work in tandem with oncologists and other therapeutic doctors but are focused on a patient's comfort, not the underlying medical condition.

A common misconception is that palliative care is given only at life's end, and it's therefore often confused with hospice care. This may be part of the fog our culture applies to anything having to do with the prospects of dying. The misunderstanding may play out in direct and subtle ways, possibly rooted in the shortsighted "gotta beat the thing" attitude discussed earlier. The result may be that palliative medicine may not play as robust a role as it should and may be so subordinated to the anticancer medical care that the major quality-of-life benefits it offers the patient—like better management of pain, nausea, appetite loss, and troubled sleeping—may get overshadowed and underutilized.

In order to effectively address the lifestyle challenges of seriously ill patients and their families, palliative care needs to be normalized and recognized as an essential puzzle piece in treating the entire patient. It needs to be made available early so its benefits can be put to use for the patient, as well as his or her family members and the entire medical team. To frame it another way, palliative medicine means Smooth River. It means quality of life. We have to better publicize it, change attitudes, and propagate its usage. It's a really good thing.

Although medical schools now offer palliative medicine training, it is still mixed up with hospice care. One study published in the *Journal of the American Heart Association* showed that "palliative care referral for heart failure patients may be suboptimal due to limited provider knowledge and misperceptions of palliative care as a service reserved for those near death."[12]

While pain management and palliative care are integral to cancer care, in our case, they could have been elevated to a higher priority level, given Marcia's wish not to suffer. Only late in the game did we become aware of the entire arsenal of pain meds available and the balance to be struck between slow-acting, time-released drugs on the one hand and fast-acting, breakthrough ones on the other. Eventually, Marcia's pain medication regimen became more fine-tuned. (More about this in chapter 15, "Dealing with Problems That Will Come.")

We also tried integrative medicine as part of a comprehensive cancer care approach. Like palliative care, integrative

---

12 Kayla Sheehan, "Nourish the Roots: The Importance of Palliative Care Education in Medical School," *Center to Advance Palliative Care*, March 25, 2020, https://www.capc.org/blog/nourish-roots-importance-palliative-care-education-medical-school/.

medicine focuses on the patient's well-being beyond the core medical disorder. It takes into account the patient's mind, spirit, and community, in addition to his or her physiology. It uses both conventional and alternative methods to facilitate the body's innate healing response, including natural approaches.

On October 14 (Day 41), we visited an integrative medicine specialist in Manhattan as part of Hospital 1's cancer management continuum. He recommended that Marcia concentrate on "big-bang-for-the-buck" foods—those that add protein and sustainable calories and do not cause sugar highs and rapid bloating—and that she walk after eating to boost her metabolism and stimulate her digestive system. Sitting or lying down after eating can make the breakdown of food more difficult. The integrative medicine specialist reviewed certain Eastern approaches like acupuncture and meditation and recommended to us the following supplements based on supportive data:

- Vitamin D3, which some studies have shown to have beneficial anticancer properties and can prolong life for those afflicted, although results are variable and inconclusive[13]
- Turkey tail (mushroom extract), which has been reported to stimulate immune function in women with breast cancer
- ProBiota Bifido, a brand of bifidobacteria, which several studies showed to have certain antitumor effects on the

---

13 Catherine Paddock, PhD, "Vitamin D May Prolong Life in People With Cancer," *Medical News Today*, June 7, 2019, https://www.medicalnewstoday.com/articles/325417.

development of cancer, possibly through the mechanisms of fermentation, biotransformation, and strengthening the intestinal barrier[14]

Trying to leave no stone unturned, we got a license from the state of New York to obtain medical marijuana to divert pain sensations, soften anxiety edges, distract attention from cancer's grip, and try to increase Marcia's appetite. Obtaining a license entailed seeing a doctor who qualified for the state marijuana program and then getting a prescription for a state-regulated dispensary to provide THC/CBT formulations in pill, vapor, spray, or distillate format. Marcia tried this for a month or two but found the effect to be too light, despite trying many THC/CBT combinations. At times, a friend delivered out-of-state recreational marijuana chocolates and gummies, which were far easier to administer and more effective, although Marcia used them sparingly. (New York has since legalized recreational marijuana.)

We gained key advice from integrative medicine, but Marcia's pancreatic cancer was just too powerful for the therapies currently available, both alternative and mainstream. Even though nothing worked to beat back the disease, we felt fulfilled that we were affirmatively touching every base we could to better Marcia's plight. And we were emotionally lifted by all the professionals who dedicate their careers and so much passion to the health and welfare of cancer patients. We were, and I remain, deeply grateful to everyone who cared for Marcia.

---

14 Wei Hongyun et al., "Antitumor Mechanisms of Bifidobacteria," *Oncology Letters*, 2018 Jul: 16(1): 3–8, https://www.ncbi.nlm.nih.gov/pmc/articles/PMC6019968/.

11. Peering Over the Edge: Heart-to-Hearts

**To the well-organized mind, death is but
the next great adventure.**

~J. K. Rowling

The first few days after Marcia's diagnosis were not Smooth
River. They were surreal, a nightmare we had to deal with
by ourselves. We had to break the news first to our family
and then figure out what it all meant. We knew the bad statistics, but we also heard of progress and some cases of stage
4 pancreatic cancer patients living well beyond a year after
diagnosis. We had optimism but remained grounded.

FOLFIRINOX chemo treatment began a few days after our
first oncology visit (Day 12), and it took awhile to adjust to
its poundings. Treatment started well enough, but the toxins
designed to kill the cancer also kill healthy cells and throw
normal bodily functions into disarray. The combatants—pancreatic cancer and high-octane chemo—fight it out, making

anarchy of your body. Already being pummeled by an array of strange invaders, the patient is left with the near-impossible task of pinpointing the sources of pain, the signposts of symptoms, and the details of side effects so that the medical professionals can try to quell the problems.

The dilemma is that this is not a linear equation where the patient says, "I have a pain," and the doctor responds, "I can fix it." There is so much biological churning going on that it's difficult to isolate the problem and therefore know how medically to tend to it. Ambiguities abound, and doctors do their best to quell the tumult, given limited remedies. Doctors would love to prescribe a solution, but the problems often have multiple hard-to-identify origins, and problems and origins are muddled together, constantly changing in nature, intensity, and character. The one constant is the turbulence running through the digestive tract, and, in Marcia's case, the creep of decay.

Trying to make sense of the physical and metaphysical disorder was a source of regular conversation. Although we spoke throughout the day, we reserved the late afternoon to have open-ended talks about her declining health and more philosophical subjects. Marcia wanted to have these discussions in our sunroom, an informal space with large windows looking out to the pleasant greenery of our backyard. It was light, airy, and open, possibly giving her some relief from the more closed-in rooms where she spent most of her time. It was a quiet, comfortable, and simple refuge devoid of technology and distraction. Although Marcia by then had to carry a vomit basin with her everywhere because an emetic attack could erupt at any time, I don't recall any incidents in our sunroom. It was almost as if that room were a sanctuary, a time-out from the turmoil, from the direct effects of the disease. It became a dedicated place for wide-ranging, honest, emotional, tough, and tender conversations, a place where we could say difficult things to each other in utter safety. Sometimes, even a slight change in the environment can adjust your outlook or at least evoke some new thinking.

So in this peaceful space, Marcia took a deep breath and reflected, eye to eye, heart to heart. While our conversations had no borders, having defined this space and dedicated time to speak helped Marcia solidify her thinking and added both calm and structure, freeing her to spend the other parts of the day on lighter matters or just get by.

An important aspect of our life talk was to leave it free-floating, without restriction or judgment. No matter how close we were as husband and wife, we ventured into subjects that were deeper than we had ever explored. We had never had to—death had never been so near. But now it was. And now, with the curtain pulled back, there was nothing to hide or withhold. I wanted her to be 100 percent comfortable. We both wanted to make sure that we covered everything. She wanted to leave this world with the sheets tucked in, the bed made, everything that we could control organized.

Marcia was exceedingly clear that she wanted transparency, not hype. Clarity was hardwired into her being. During our life talks, she said several times that she was too young to die, that the cancer had made her life expectancy shorter than the norm. Imminent death, especially when you thought you had decades of life left, is a lonely experience. It involves profound mental processing, fits and starts, and lots of falls before you can arrive at a new, imperfect equilibrium. Before cancer struck, we had fully expected to spend a long time together, take in adventures, explore new areas of interest, solidify the many cross-cultural pursuits we had staked out, and just enjoy what we had, especially our growing family.

Marcia's wanting to understand how the next few months might roll out and to delve into the possibility of dying—and all its hard-to-get-your-mind-around ramifications—eased our way and lifted an otherwise unbearable weight. Her innate need for order and preparation unlocked us both from the grip of fear, self-pity, and emotional inaction. In the movie *A Beautiful Day in the Neighborhood*, Tom Hanks, playing Mister Rogers, observes, "Anything mentionable is manageable." While at first it was uncomfortable for her to say and me to hear, by putting into words her inner thoughts, distress, and lost dreams, Marcia softened the scary loose ends left to the imagination. She made me a better listener and dissolved my mental blocks in facing the prospect of losing her. The more we talked, the more manageable the emotional morass became for both of us. In real time, we were learning the process of dying and therefore the art of living.

Immediately after the diagnosis, Marcia assembled a library of books about death and dying and how to live a meaningful life. She had already experienced loss, having buried both her parents and a brother. Back then, Harold S. Kushner's *When Bad Things Happen to Good People* and its message had resonated with her: that bad things that befall us may have no meaning, but "we can redeem these tragedies from sense-lessness by imposing meaning on them." Now other books became important, too, in helping Marcia see that her situation was not unique, that others had experienced premature death, many under even more abrupt circumstances, such as heart attacks and aneurysms, automobile accidents, and acts of violence—when life shuts off in an instant, when there is no time to prepare, no chance to say goodbye. While Marcia wanted to live far longer, she knew she was blessed by having already led an accomplished life. Her reading list is assembled in Appendix 2. These and other references are listed on www.smoothriver.org.

Before cancer, Marcia had expected smooth sailing for a long time, to bask in the joy of seeing her grandson growing up and the birth of her granddaughter, to immerse in family experiences, to laugh and cry with family and friends, to get lost in new unknowns, and to ride the wave of life into the distant sunset. Who thinks about getting pancreatic cancer other than out of Woody Allen paranoia? It was a contingency we had never considered but we now had to play out. And on the uncertain playing field, with the stakes so high and the moment of truth upon her, she came to the realization that she had already been blessed by having led a full life. That was deeply freeing.

During our dedicated life talks, we discussed her dreams, our family, our new Florida house gambit, her dying younger than we would want, whatever came to her mind. She mentioned often how she wanted me to be happy and find a new balance after she was gone and so I could look after our sons and their families. She was concerned about their welfare, the impact her death would have on them. They were no longer children where the loss of a parent can imprint itself in complicated, lifelong ways. But she was still their mother who was leaving them too soon. What would that mean? We talked and talked. And I promised that I would try to take on her personality in my dealings with them. That is, to reflect her calm, softness, and understanding, to become their friend. It turned out that I've become part her in dealing with everyone and everything.

During our talks, she took us to uncharted places. She wanted to explore the surprisingly fleeting nature of life and what the nothingness of death feels like. These were hard, painful topics to talk about because it meant that Marcia had crossed the Rubicon and would be gone. You can delve into these matters in the abstract and surmise some answers, but when you are put in a place where death is your neighbor and extinction is near, the unimaginable suddenly becomes imaginable, words give voice to the ineffable, and voids are filled with elements detectable by senses you didn't think you had.

So, sitting on our sunroom couch, facing each other with moistened eyes and heavy hearts, we wandered into the nothingness of death. We touched its bare, jagged walls; smelled its damp muskiness; and adjusted to its darkness to look around and be where we were not supposed to be. We were trying to talk about the inanimate quality of being dead as if we both were dead and alive at the same time, separating ourselves into two beings, one lifeless and one an observer. As observers, we came to understand ourselves as being stilled of life. We did this together so Marcia would not have to go there alone, at least not yet. We came to understand that we would have no thoughts or feelings when we were gone. That we become part of the earth and return to the inexplicable cosmos from whence we came. But before that happened, we lived and we loved. We touched other people and other people touched us. We struggled and strived. Sometimes we succeeded but often fell short. We scratched and we clawed to rise above our limitations and experience new places and new people and bring new insights and meaning to our family, friends, and others we knew. We tried to do good, maybe made an ailing person smile, came to someone's aid, helped solve a problem, guided our children and grandchildren.

We came to understand that before we pass, we have shed seeds of ourselves all over the place. Some have taken root and influenced another directly. Some may have a more attenuated impact. Some will scatter to the wind and not land on anyone or anything. But, I told Marcia, virtually all of her seeds had landed on me, and while she would enter nonexistence first, her goodness has made me a better person and will always guide me. We both understood that everyone will enter nothingness. However one views this inevitability—as an inanimate end; as a gateway to heaven, hell, or the hereafter; or as something else and unknown—we agreed it is connected to the life we have led and the seeds we have sown. And these seeds will grow again.

Another tender subject was the actual process of dying. One day, in the flat light of an early-winter afternoon, she looked straight into my eyes and asked, "Rich, how am I going to die?

What's it going to be like? What should I expect?" We both read up on the physiological breaking down of the body. She read that at a certain point a dying person has to say good-bye and take the final steps by herself. She said that I would have to let her go. The finality of this was shattering, but her strong will to explore the path to the end was so Marcia. She was addressing subjects we shrink from but now needed to be examined.

I said I wasn't certain of the process, but I imagined I would be by her side physically to the end and that we would be part of each other in spirit way past then. I would comfort her and keep her company every moment, while she was awake and while she was asleep, until the last one. We would be together, and she would know it until she would not know it any longer. And right then, as she crossed the divide, I would be there to take her in when she was no longer able to breathe. And then, by way of some ethereal transference, I would breathe for her and carry on.

And that was exactly what happened.

12. Keeping Your Eye on the Medical Road and Both Hands on the Wheel

Action may not always bring happiness, but there is no happiness without action.

~William James

Given all that was at stake, we wanted to find the right medical team and just defer completely to it. We wanted to surrender and trust that they would take care of us completely so that we could tend to all the nonmedical affairs.

I have enormous respect for the health-care system and those who work in it. But the system is a massive enterprise. Doctors, nurses, and other personnel do their best to treat each patient on a personalized basis, but the sheer volume of people they see and the workload they carry made it impossible for health-care workers to meet our idealistic expectations, plus everybody is human. Health-care workers have their own professional and personal stressors like everyone else.

We wanted to be exceedingly careful to defer to the professionals we chose, to respect their expertise, and not to be do-it-yourselfers or second-guessers. But we came to understand that we had jobs to do in assisting the fine people treating Marcia. We found it important to do our homework ahead of appointments, maintain our logs, prepare lists of questions, and be respectful of our providers' time, knowing other patients needed their attention as well. Maintaining a good rapport with one's providers is wise personal policy. It promotes a more rewarding experience and recognizes the good works of those taking care of you.

Years ago, I invented a few homemade, commonsense laws of human conduct based on my own experience under pressure. They turned out to be particularly valuable to us as we made our way through the white waters of pancreatic cancer.

The Law of Self-Responsibility

This law means that when you look at a situation, it's best to make sure you have taken care of everything that would be reasonably expected of you and try to stretch into new functions you could be handling. You don't want to be pointing fingers or come across as unreasonable or entitled.

In cancer world, I applied the law of self-responsibility to keep a check on myself so that I wouldn't slough off tasks I could perform. This guideline is not meant to be a push to do things that are beyond one's means or abilities, but rather a gentle reminder not to shirk responsibilities and opportunities to take certain actions. It pays to be vigilant and active in caring for a patient and yourself. The risk in not being an active team member is that clinicians can inadvertently overlook some things or be too busy to timely perform certain tasks you can do just as easily. Relying on others for something you can comfortably do could erode goodwill that can otherwise serve the patient. Keeping a log of key medical and life events and an up-to-date listing of medications (and side effects), prompting doctors and their assistants for prescription renewals and to follow up on test results, and getting to appointments on time and coming prepared to make the most of each visit were just part of the responsibility Marcia and I took on in participating in her care.

The Law of Compassion

In cancer world, the law of self-responsibility should not be *mistakenly* used to blame yourself for the cancer or not catching it earlier than you did.[15] In our case, the diagnosis turned us, for a short period, into detectives seeking clues or warning signs that we might have overlooked: "If only Marcia saw a doctor months earlier when she was sleeping more than eight hours a day," or "If only she took more notice of increasing fatigue." It didn't take long for us to realize that this woulda-coulda-shoulda syndrome is distracting and dangerous. It can draw you into a continuous cycle of self-rebuke and set a slippery slope descending the depressive scale. The fact is what is done is done, and we can only go forward.

Compounding the dangers of associating past conduct with your present condition is a cultural instinct that may subtly

---

15 Rev. Percy McCray Jr., "Is This Cancer My Fault?" *Cancer Treatment Centers of America*, September 4, 2019, https://www.cancercenter.com/community/blog/2019/09/is-this-cancer-my-fault.

play out by judging cancer victims for failing to prevent the disease. Psychologically, many people opt for the simplicity of finding fault with a patient in contributing to his or her own predicament rather than dealing with messy realities. Ascribing fault may feel like it provides an answer and adds some cognitive clarity, but it is unfounded. The reality is far more complex and subtle. Yes, there may be family history, and yes, there are risk factors that can be determinative. But for most of us, the fact is we will never truly know why some fall ill and others don't, why some have engaged in certain conduct and others not. We have no choice but to put compassion first and to live with ambiguities, unanswered questions, troubling truths, and even lifestyle choices a patient may have made that seem ill advised.

For the patient's trusted group of confidants, not only does none of this matter, but the actualities of terminal illness reveal how superficial it is to center on anything except the patient's well-being. There is no room for blame, no right to judge, no point in being critical. This is a time for love and personal growth. Period.

The Law of Self-Interest

Doctors operate on top of a hierarchy whereby they leverage their experience and expertise over a broad team of other health-care professionals, such as physician assistants, registered nurses, nurse practitioners, administrative assistants, and other staff. The team needs to enter a lot of information into medical records and patient portals; order, refill, and keep track of many drugs; and coordinate treatment logistics for each patient, on top of research, teaching, and administrative work. Clinicians are only human, and sometimes, things are not followed up or correctly recorded, and glitches happen with software and online connections. Even if things work perfectly, patients and their loved ones play a critical advocacy role.

Enter what I call the Law of Self-Interest. It is not meant to be a license to be self-absorbed or to disregard the rights of others. It is simply a recognition that a party whose interests are being tested has the intrinsic and unique motivation to find ways to advance them. It's another prompt to diplomatically stand up for yourself and not be inhibited. Many times, we had to remind doctors and their assistants to phone in new prescriptions to our pharmacy, to respond to certain questions we had, or to obtain and help us interpret test results. Another example was my hunting down, as a last resort, the human form of dog dewormers, however way-out this measure might have been. (More on this in chapter 16.)

The Law of Inevitability

This law guards against procrastination. It provides that if something is inevitable, take care of it sooner rather than later. Assuming that you have carefully thought out some course of action and there are no preceding conditions to executing it—whether or not the subject is medically related—putting off action can fester in you, clutter your mind, and logjam other things you need to do. You don't want something hanging over you when you need to free your mind and time for the things that really matter. More importantly, you don't want to delay doing what may seem awkward or unpleasant when it comes to your medical care when time is not on your side.

After Marcia and I resolved to switch oncologists, we didn't wait. And we did it in a way that guaranteed a safe landing with the new oncologist and preserved the relationship with the first one. We could have gotten stuck in inertia by deferring that difficult conversation. Taking care of it saved us time and unnecessary mental overhang while freeing us to do what needed to be done.

The Law of Gratitude

We learned that even though we were in crisis, we could conduct ourselves the way we always did: by putting ourselves in the shoes of the other. We always felt that life is bigger than ourselves, and now this point was made abundantly clear due to our dependence on countless health-care personnel. The perspective of appreciating others helped us create friendly relationships with our caregivers and reminded us of who we were as people.

It was not our nature to react to urgencies with uncontrolled abandon and become too hotheaded to handle. Marcia liked people, as do I, and we became attached to nearly everyone who cared for her. We believe this sincerity was reciprocated. But even so, we always looked for ways to express our appreciation. We often brought donuts, bagels, or other gifts for the nurses, the security staff, and other personnel just to show that we valued them and that they were special. We even had flowers delivered to Dr. B's assistant. (As is in business, assistants are the ones who usually get things done.) Showing appreciation for everyone in the chain of command, at every level, in every function, not only pays dividends, it's the right thing to do. Marcia's kind and thankful demeanor—and her out-of-the-blue, funny one-liners—no matter how she was feeling, certainly made caring for her more pleasant for all medical personnel.

Now, some other practical gleanings derived from our experience in the trenches.

Navigating Online Portals

Nowadays, virtually all hospitals offer some online information system to be used by the patient and his or her advocates. They've become even more important in the increasingly present, noncontact environments. Setting online portals can be a bit of a chore, especially for those not computer literate, but once done, the portal provides an effective communication medium. Sometimes we interacted with our clinicians via the portal, sometimes outside of it by phone, text, or email. Sometimes we had no choice but to use it, like when seeing test results that were recorded online. When we wanted to keep an organized written record of our asks to the medical professionals, posting messages online was helpful. Sometimes we used it to repeat a request to fill a prescription, change an appointment, or let our doctor know of a new symptom or drug reaction. We tried to economize our communications so as not to be a burden, but posting friendly reminders on the portal worked well for all of us.

Often, we uploaded nonclinical notes and photos reflecting our Life Plan, such as how Marcia fared on our trips to Florida or how we enjoyed a meal at a restaurant. We hoped that by broadening the scope of our discourse, our doctors would have a more well-rounded picture of Marcia and how she was doing. One point was to pass on how the cancer, chemos, medications, and side effects were impacting her. Another was to demonstrate the broader life of a patient, a core element of the perspective provided by Smooth River thinking.

Some functions offered by hospital portals include:

- Appointments—List of upcoming and past appointments
- Medical information—Patient information, such as allergies, medications, prior surgeries, and medical conditions
- Messages—From and to your doctor
- Test and lab results—Posted by your doctor, radiology professionals, or lab personnel
- Resources—Search for information within the hospital's online library or other online resources
- Billing—Insurance information and status of outstanding bills
- Records—Such as medical proxies, living wills, do-not-resuscitate orders, and other legal documentation

Understanding Test Results and Getting Professional Context

Often, the radiology or pathology departments posted CT scan and CA 19–9 tumor marker test results online before we had a chance to speak with our oncologist for context. A doctor's preference would generally be to first discuss the results with a patient and not have the patient try to interpret them in a vacuum. But the information system may be too complex to manage the wishes of every doctor.

Several times, we saw negative CT scan and CA 19–9 results before our doctor was able to explain their meaning. When we did speak, qualifications and nuance would be conveyed to underscore that we shouldn't necessarily jump to any conclusions regarding the test results. But the negative trendline was obvious, and without any positive data, the prognosis clarified how much time Marcia had—even if the doctors refrained from making predictions. We saw the writing on the wall. We hoped for some reversal. We hoped for any good news—even neutral news—but in its absence held firm to our Smooth River vision, which kept us steady.

In-Hospital Doctor Visits and Rotations

Marcia was admitted to Lawrence Hospital in Bronxville from January 3–5, 2020 (Days 122–124) due to a sudden and dangerous drop in blood pressure, and then again from January 16–19 (Days 135–138). She entered NY-Presbyterian on January 19 (Day 138) and stayed until January 26 (Day 145) to be treated for internal bleeding. Finally, because of a variety of biological breakdowns, we had to take an ambulance on January 30 (Day 149) to Lawrence, where Marcia stayed until the end, February 10 (Day 160).

Hospitals are remarkably organized places, even with understandable breakdowns here and there. There are coteries of doctors, nurses, and other clinicians making rounds while an attending physician, nurse, and other staff are usually assigned to each patient, and when the assigned personnel go on break, others cover.

A shift change involves the rotating staff spending time with one another to pass along notes, observations, and patient status. Several times a day, nurses and doctors meet at centralized nursing stations. Among other things, they review one another's cases and overall conditions, sharing information, helping one another, and seeking to make improvements, all pursuant to hospital standards and protocols.

As an outsider observing all this, I found the commitment inspiring. It's busy, sometimes messy, sometimes chaotic, but always impressive, exceptions and imperfections and all. What can one say about the throngs of professionals who take care of us with such dedication, skill, and heart, many commuting for hours by subway or car, juggling their own family and personal needs? The atmosphere is far from the serenity of a place of worship or a babbling brook. But it, too, is pretty divine.

Among the many disciplines making rounds are the generalist doctors (attending physicians, sometimes called hospitalists) who oversee a patient's care and specialists in various areas like gastroenterology, hematology (blood), nutrition, palliative care, interventional radiologists, and physical and occupational therapy. Chaplains, personal care, transport staff, and food service personnel are among the other professionals whose office is the hospital.

So many people cycle through, it's hard to keep track of everyone, their concentrations, their names, and their contact information. We found it useful to get business cards from the doctors and otherwise take careful notes. In each room, there was typically an erasable whiteboard with the contact info for the attending physician and shift nurse. Not knowing when medical personnel would show up, I wrote my name and cell number prominently on the whiteboard in case I went out for a bite or was doing work in an open area or lounge while Marcia was napping.

None of this is to say that we didn't encounter some issues with hospital personnel. Based on the advice of radiation oncologists (rad-oncs), we opted for some palliative radiation toward the end to relieve Marcia's pain and stem internal bleeding. But during a critical moment in Marcia's last week, a different doctor who didn't know my wife, our bond, or our Smooth River philosophy sought to impose his own values and opinions on Marcia when I wasn't in her room and persuade her against our symptom management course. I had to explain to this doctor that although these were Marcia's decisions to make, being on high levels of Fentanyl pain medication and other drugs, her judgment was somewhat cloudy and I needed to be part of the discussions to help her balance the many factors that affect decision-making. After hearing about this incident, our rad-onc agreed with me and told me to refer to her anyone trying to steer Marcia or me in another direction.

Pain, nausea, and constipation continued to be major issues. The whiteboard in Marcia's room featured a one-to-ten pain scale with a happy face at one and very sad face at ten. We recorded pain scales several times a day, often on a high number with a grumpy face. A nurse cannot administer pain medication or other drugs within a hospital without a doctor's order. There were times when we had to wait inordinately long for a prescription to be written or filled by the hospital pharmacy. It's not a perfect system, and managing Marcia's pain was an issue. It was finally brought under control during her last two months when strong preventative maintenance, extended-release meds were prescribed.

Throughout the swirling currents of activity, Marcia remained a gracious and sociable host for all medical personnel. Just as she did in her professional and personal worlds, she made hospital workers feel at ease, always looking for the opportunity to make them smile, or better yet, laugh. Maybe that was why many clinicians left us their cell numbers and texted us to ask how Marcia was doing. We were so in awe of all these people who devote their lives to helping others.

13. Preparing for the End

**We all die. The goal isn't to live forever,
the goal is to create something that will.**
~Chuck Palahniuk

When life fades, a tide of emotions collides with hard practicalities. One needs the freedom to experience raw pain and sorrow but find the discipline to keep afloat and even help your loved ones do so. All the while, the world keeps turning, reminding you that actions need to be taken and documents signed. Preparing for the end involves shedding our earthly veneer and "going vulnerable" in expressing our innermost thoughts, but with a pen in hand to protect your and your loved ones' interests.

Coming Together As a Family
Integral to Marcia's coming to terms with the likelihood of dying was her getting comfortable with the idea that her family would be whole after she passed. We were fortunate that

our immediate family carried no major interpersonal issues, although like all families, there is always room to soften the edges. There were disagreements and arguments, of course. Long marriages and the joyous chaos of family life are like that. To ease Marcia's concerns, we made clear that we would be brokenhearted and deeply empty without her but that she would be leaving us with a trove of gifts to carry forward as a loving family who has one another's backs. Some of Marcia's gifts included her admonitions to keep things simple, not to get bogged down in detail, shock-absorb the hits, and not let our egos get in the way of embracing one another. It was reassuring for Marcia to understand that she was the one to provide us with the medicine to heal and the tools to go on productively. Nearly every day, I let her know that I would be more Marcia-like in helping our family and interacting with everyone else. In her life, she had accomplished so much and somehow had made it all look so straightforward and easy. I'm still learning the benefits of simplicity and efficiency from her.

Throughout her illness, but especially as the end neared, each of my sons spent more time with Marcia, sometimes alone, often as a family. We liked just being together. We didn't even have to speak. We all knew we were soaking in every second of her presence, praying for some way to stretch out the time so our being all together would never wind down. I cried to myself often just watching these beautiful gatherings, knowing it would all come to an end soon.

So despite whatever tiffs and bruised feelings that existed, the gravity of Marcia's illness drew us together like a magnet. It was so important for Marcia to know that our feelings for one another were deep and durable and she could have mental peace when the time came to say goodbye. After all that she had done for us, we knew she deserved to bathe in eternal well-being while here and in the hereafter.

Other families may have more complicated issues involving many emotional crosscurrents. There is no way to make light of them. They can manifest deep wounds. Yet, however painful the issues may be, the imminent death of a loved one may provide opportunities to rise above them or at least view them in a different way, even if just for a short while. I've come to see that so many arguments among people seem based on an injury to our sense of honor.

Conflict-resolution experts often advise putting a dispute into writing, which tends to crystallize loose elements of discord in a form that can then be attended to. One fruitful goal is to channel emotional issues into a tangible project that may be addressed in a mutually respectful manner whereby everyone comes together for the benefit of the patient. Unifying around a common purpose can heal long-held grievances, stimulate new beginnings, and untie psychological knots.

Serious health situations can be a cathartic moment to reach a new accord for reconciliation and forgiveness. Although pure love and altruism should be the motivator, there are good reasons to rise above family conflict and find a calmer altitude, to settle issues, or just let them pass and evaporate. This is the time to liberate yourself, shed the armor, expose your heart, and express it. Grant your loved one the immense relief of knowing that he or she is departing a family as one, or at least dedicated to making the effort to heal prior wounds. This by itself is heavenly.

Legal Documents

Well in advance of getting sick and in preparation for whatever life threw at us, Marcia and I had gotten key documents together years ago. One of her high-profile clients had recommended a reasonably priced lawyer to draw up wills, living wills, and medical proxies.

We might have revised these documents once or twice since then, as laws had changed, but for a long time, we honestly had no idea what they said. Now, faced with the odds of Marcia's early departure, she and I asked a new lawyer to review them. Besides tax matters that will vary from person to person and state to state, there are important decisions to be made in terms of who gets what. There is the material aspect of dispensing value to beneficiaries, but also emotional issues involved; bequests can be packed with meaning. Marcia liked to say in relation to many business and personal challenges: "It's not so much about the thing itself, but what the thing represents," meaning whatever the issue is, there is usually a deeper, unresolved conflict that gets scraped open. So deciding on a will's provisions is far more than a legal exercise. With a trusted, experienced professional, it should involve a careful assessment of what bequests you would like to make, the possible impacts of the gifts on the intended beneficiaries, financial planning, emotional intelligence, choice of executors and trustees, and an array of tangible and intangible factors that will leave a mark. The consequences of an uneven distribution among siblings and other close relations can be severe. Yet thoughtful bestowals can change lives and otherwise make a difference.

A living will refers to a legally enforceable writing that spells out a patient's preferences in regard to certain life-extending measures if and when a patient is no longer able to express them. In a living will, depending upon the state law involved, a person can decide if he or she wishes to be given life-sustaining treatments in the event of a terminal condition, such as inserting a feeding tube or using heart-lung machines, ventilators, and other medical equipment that may extend life but offer no cure. Without such a directive, families may have to obtain court orders to make critical medical decisions. According to the American Bar Association, doctors can refuse to follow living will provisions if they have an objection of conscience or consider your wishes medically inappropriate, but in that case, they must transfer the patient to a health-care provider who will follow the orders.[16]

A health-care proxy is a durable power of attorney specifically designed to cover medical treatment. In it, you appoint a person and grant him or her the authority to make medical decisions for you in the event you are unable to express your preferences. Most commonly, this situation occurs either because you are unconscious or because your mental state is such that you do not have the legal capacity to make your own decisions.

Marcia and I made sure to upload these documents to the online portals of our hospitals, in addition to providing hard

16 Charles Sabatino, "Myths and Facts About Health Care Advance Directives," The American Bar Association Commission on Law and Aging, *BIFOCAL* 37, no. 1 (September–October 2015), https://www.american-bar.org/groups/law_aging/publications/bifocal/vol_37/issue_1_october2015/myths_and_facts_advance_directives/.

copies. We wanted to avoid ambiguity in the event one of the conditions set forth in the documents was triggered.

An enlightened nonprofit organization called Aging with Dignity composed a thoughtful document called Five Wishes® that serves as a legally binding advance directive in most states and is available in more than twenty-five languages. In contrast to the legalese of conventional forms, it is written in user-friendly, familiar language and addresses a range of end-of-life matters, including providing instructions by the patient for the medical care desired, the comfort levels the patient wants to achieve, how the patient wants to be regarded by loved ones, and wishes the patient wants his or her loved ones to know. Marcia and I did not use the Five Wishes® legal directive but did use the document as a foundation for composing her final wishes, as discussed in chapter 19.

Another excellent resource is Advance Care Planning: Health Care Directives, developed by the National Institute on Aging, a private, nonprofit organization with a mission to safeguard and affirm the human dignity of those who face the challenges and opportunities of aging or serious illness.

Given Marcia's situation, she chose not to include an organ donation directive, but this is another legal aspect to end-of-life planning.

In regard to all of the above, and every other item in this book that touches on professional matters, it is a good idea to consult with a trusted lawyer, doctor, or other qualified expert.

Insurance and Benefits

Marcia did have life insurance and 401(k) benefits, which were important to revisit in terms of rethinking who the beneficiaries were and making sure everything was still effective. There may be tax reasons or life reasons to shift the beneficiaries from those originally designated or to amend certain other provisions. Here, too, a trusted professional should be consulted.

Within the first two months of her diagnosis, I almost fainted when we got a letter saying that Marcia's life insurance would lapse in a few weeks because we accidentally had not paid the annual premium. Thinking the impending lapse was another sign of things falling apart, I nervously arranged to make the payment on the insurer's website that same day. It was still within the reinstatement period, but the close call wasn't Smooth River. Better to check in advance on the effectiveness of life insurance, retirement, and other benefits that spring from your or your loved one's passing.

14. Discovering Spiritual Beauty within the Storm

Life is truly lived in the moments of simplicity!
~Avijeet Das

Taking care of Marcia and understanding that she felt embarrassed by her dependence on me, even while accepting there was no choice, was a profound experience. After a lifetime of tending to the professional and personal needs of others, her vulnerability now was an excruciating threshold for my proud wife to cross. It broke my heart to see her so defenseless, but at the same time, I loved the trust we had in each other. It was gratifying on so many levels to help her live and take care of all the little things that sanctified her remaining time, our remaining time.

There is something beautiful about tending to your wife in an elemental way. Vanity, materialism, and privacy dissolve and create new intimacy. At the edge of life, one's being is reduced to its quintessence. Emotion rises to heights that defy description, and it is love that gives you the fortitude and guidance to carry on. With death approaching, there is no time to get hung up about inhibitions or hold back.

Drying Marcia's hair when she couldn't became a deeply moving experience. After I helped her out of the shower onto a small chair, I would stand behind her, watching her face in the mirror and her frail body from behind, put the blow-dryer on low, hold it in one hand, and slowly pat her hair dry with my other, separating out the strands and feeling her soft hair flow through my fingers. That was the sensuous ritual I observed before carefully introducing a brush to ride down the slopes of her silky hair. Throughout, our eyes kept meeting in the mirror, and volumes of words flowed unspoken.

This was only the start of tending to Marcia's hygiene. She deteriorated so quickly that I needed to help her shower, move her to and from the toilet and, toward the end, a commode. She was ashamed to disrobe in front of me because of how thin she appeared. She warned me that I might be scared to look at her naked. But there would be no separation between us. Whatever condition she was in, I was in. I became her, but with the physical strength to do what needed to be done.

This intense, waning phase of our long connection, when all there was, was trust and truth, called up everything she and I had shared and brought into view the divergent tracks laid out for us. It is right here before our paths would split, at the transition between life and death, that our entire existence from birth flashed back before us, and all our experiences, good and bad, found transcendent meaning.

Yet through it all, I watched Marcia shift in bed from one position to another and ambulate by taking one small, unsteady step after another, often bracing against a dresser or table and, in the last few days, moving with the aid of a walker. I saw her trudge up and down the stairs sometimes on her feet, sometimes on her rear, before we installed a stair lift. I watched her wheel an IV pole to the hospital bathroom and through the hallways to take short walks. I watched her daily rituals to create order and tidiness on her night table and direct the rest of us to unclutter her room. I watched how she washed her face and applied simple fragrances to retain an air of dignity. I listened to the waterfall spills of her mind, always progressing, always thinking ahead, always organized. She moved in the big picture, seemingly at a higher altitude with lower atmospheric pressure than many of us who get stuck in the tar of everyday affairs.

Albert Einstein once said, "Life is like riding a bicycle. To keep your balance, you must keep moving." Throughout the entire ordeal, Marcia never stopped moving. She never got off her bike, even when her abilities were declining, from being able to walk and stand to only being able to sit or lie prone, from being able to eat, talk, text, and laugh to only being able to sip ice chips and move her eyes. Throughout it all, there was unspeakable beauty in every muscle contraction, every turn of her cheek, every effort to smile, every twinkle in her eye. Life and love at their most primal levels—soaring in meaning when there is nothing else and the end is near—can be quite exhilarating, made more so by shedding all thoughts other than those of the moment.

The point: hug your kids, cuddle your spouse, embrace your relatives and friends, accept yourself. It will all vanish someday.

15. Dealing with Problems That Will Come

The problem is not that there are problems.
The problem is expecting otherwise and thinking
that having problems is a problem.
~Theodore Isaac Rubin

Pancreatic cancer is a tsunami. Together with its poisonous chemo counterpoint, it creates mayhem on several fronts. We had to learn on the job and, with the aid of our medical team, deal with each problem as it arose. There are textbook responses to many core problems, but actually handling them in real time requires a more brass tacks, improvised approach.

Chemo Brain

The American Cancer Society describes chemo brain as a mental cloudiness, a cancer-related cognitive impairment. Chemo patients can have trouble remembering things, finishing tasks, or concentrating. I believe it impacted Marcia, but I'm 100 percent certain it hit me, even though I was not in the defined class. That was because in addition to the intangible heaviness of everything circulating around us, there were so many to-do lists to keep, appointments to track, drugs to take, people to get back to, things to take care of. The problem is when you're having chemo or tending to a loved one who is, you can't operate with the same efficiency you're used to. This by itself can leave more items unfinished, but on top of that, it's frustrating not to be as productive and sharp as normal.

Our way of handling it was humor. We could take care of priorities with checklists, Outlook appointments, and the part of memory that resonates when a need is high. With some items we ranked as less important and let slip, we just cut ourselves some slack and laughed at trying to run while shoulder deep in a pool of water. There was just too much resistance.

Medical professionals may have more precise ways to manage chemo brain, but our Smooth River mindset helped to lighten its effects by clarifying the bigger picture.

Pain

Marcia made it clear from the start that she was going to meet the challenge and would take all reasonable actions to beat back the cancer, but she wanted her pain mitigated. Pain management is very tricky, and it's very much trial and error. Pain can come from several sources. In Marcia's case, it came from the pancreatic tumor growing and pressing against her stomach and the nerve endings in the stomach lining. As the pain was often more intense while lying down, Marcia opted to sit up when awake and to sleep with her upper body propped up by pillows.

It is nearly impossible to maintain a good quality of life when besieged by pain. When a patient is suffering, doing anything is a hassle. It's difficult to be with anyone, even family. Some doctors may be hesitant in prescribing pain medication for fear of making a patient too loopy. Regrettably, we found out late in the process that there was ample room to medicate Marcia safely and improve her experience without knocking her out.

When over-the-counter remedies like Tylenol and ibuprofen don't work, opioids are the primary tools to treat pain from pancreatic cancer and other severe conditions. Opioids work by binding to opioid receptors in our nervous system and, via several complex chemical processes, interfering with the ability of molecules called neurotransmitters to transmit the sensation of pain. Some patients fear taking (and some doctors fear giving) opioid-based pain drugs because that may lead to addiction or cause unwanted changes in their mental state. But taking medicine for cancer pain rarely leads to addiction or misuse and is a whole different ballgame. Responding to a five-year study published in the *Journal of the National Cancer Institute*, the doctors who authored the piece wrote, "The findings raise concerns about whether opioid prescribing legislation and guidelines intended for the noncancer population are being applied inappropriately to patients with cancer and survivors."[17]

---

17 NCI staff, "Are Cancer Patients Getting the Opioids They Need to Control Pain?" National Cancer Institute at the National Institutes of Health, September 16, 2020 https://www.cancer.gov/news-events/cancer-currents-blog/2020/opioids-cancer-pain-oncologists-decreasing-prescriptions.

Several experts have concluded that in our greater society, chronic pain "is largely underdiagnosed, often undertreated, and expected to increase as the American population ages."[18] Because of the potential for abuse and addiction, many clinicians hesitate to prescribe potentially beneficial agents. Even in the world of cancer care, where addiction is not a material concern, doctors can underutilize available medications, leaving patients in physical agony on top of existential worries of impending death. One prospective study of 3,123 patients with invasive cancer of the breast, prostate, colon/rectum, or lung showed that one-third of the patients had inadequate analgesic (painkiller) prescribing.[19]

With the introduction of longer-lasting opioid formulations in the late 1990s, there are now more flexible and effective tools in managing pain. Relief is more readily achievable by finding the right balance of extended-release and immediate-release meds.

A quick primer:

Extended-release opioids are indicated for the management of severe pain when a continuous, around-the-clock analgesic is needed. They are slow-release, long-lasting drugs that act for twelve, twenty-four, or even seventy-two hours and are supposed to lower the baseline level of pain. They work through a controlled release of the active agent for relatively consistent and

---

18 Michael J. Brennan, "Update on Prescription Extended-Release Opioids and Appropriate Patient Selection," *Journal of Multidisciplinary Healthcare*, 2013, 6:265–280, https://www.ncbi.nlm.nih.gov/pmc/articles/PMC3726523/.

19 Michael J. Fisch et al., "Prospective, Observational Study of Pain and Analgesic Prescribing in Medical Oncology Outpatients with Breast, Colorectal, Lung, or Prostate cancer," *Journal of Clinical Oncology*, 2012; 30:1980–1988. [PMC free article] [PubMed] [Google Scholar].

prolonged relief with lower concentration and fewer peak-to-trough fluctuations. The intention is to take them in advance of pain, staying ahead of it, rather than reacting to urgent attacks with immediate-release drugs. The ones that Marcia took were:

- OxyContin (the time-release version of oxycodone) pills. Taken twice daily.
- Fentanyl transdermal patches (changed every seventy-two hours, but the frequency can be customized). Only in Marcia's final months was Fentanyl prescribed; it would have been helpful earlier on.

Immediate-release opioids act quicker and stronger, but are for short-term episodes, having a clinical effect for about three to six hours. Even so, these breakthrough drugs still take a short while to provide relief, leaving the patients writhing until they take effect. They also can produce a sugar high—a spate of relief—and then make a quick exit. By themselves, they were inadequate to tend to the kind of intense, long-lasting pain that afflicted Marcia and impacts other patients. Marcia was prescribed:

- Oxycodone—the active ingredient in a number of narcotic pain medications, including OxyContin
- Oxycodone acetaminophen (Percocet)
- Tramadol (Ultram)
- Hydromorphone (Dilaudid)

All opioids are controlled substances and must of course be taken under the supervision of a doctor.

Opioid analgesics are categorized as either weak (e.g., codeine, hydrocodone plus acetaminophen, and tramadol) or strong (e.g., oxycodone, hydromorphone, morphine, Fentanyl, and oxymorphone).[20]

Pain is usually measured by the patient being asked to rate the pain's intensity based on the ubiquitous zero-to-ten scale, as previously mentioned. Zero means no pain, one to three means mild pain, four to seven is considered moderate pain, and eight and above signals severe pain. Often, Marcia reported pain above seven.

Being subjective and simple, the pain scale has obvious limitations. Although it seeks to translate patient sensations with some standardization, it overlooks vital details, like whether the pain is tolerable, how it interferes with everyday functions, and other qualitative features.

However pain is measured, Marcia felt undermedicated during the first four months—up to about Day 120. At first, she was given Tramadol and Percocet. Tramadol is a pill to help relieve moderate to moderately severe pain. Percocet is oxycodone with Tylenol. The first time she was upped to something with sufficient potency and around-the-clock action was on Day 124. It was two days after she had collapsed in our home due to dangerously low blood pressure and was admitted to Lawrence Hospital. That was when she was given a seventy-two-hour, 25-microgram Fentanyl transdermal patch. The dosage would increase substantially in the coming weeks until the right levels were reached.

---

20 Andrea M. Trescot et al., "Opioid Pharmacology," *Pain Physician*, 2008;11:S133–S153, https://pubmed.ncbi.nlm.nih.gov/18443637/.

Marcia and I learned pain management under fire; her pain was sometimes so searing that she compared it to labor during childbirth. I wish we had known from the start about the entire arsenal of pain medications available. I wish we had known about the critical balance between extended- and immediate-release medications and the elastic adjustments that could have been made to keep Marcia comfortable. Because so many factors influence pain and the sensation can overwhelm a patient's ability to manage his or her cancer care experience, it would seem appropriate that the palliative medicine team play an early and leading role in cancer care, laying out all the options and actively discussing all available medications with the patient. Studies have found that palliative medicine is underutilized due to insufficient provider knowledge. But I have to wonder whether palliative care, with its soft "treat the entire patient" approach, is overshadowed by the more muscular "beat the cancer" mentality prevalent in our society. Medicine is at its best when all options and considerations are put on the table for the patient to consider.

Pretty late in the game, we learned that the trick was to be in front of the pain and dull it before it acted up, but when it did, to take the quick-release breakthrough meds to handle those spikes. If all you are doing is taking breakthrough meds, you would be putting out fires all day and raising your tolerance levels, which thereby requires increasingly higher dosages. Optimally, you can raise the extended-release medication level to where it is controlling most of the pain before it happens and then leave some gunpowder for attacks with the quick-release drugs.

While Marcia was an inpatient at NY-Presbyterian (Days 138–145), one smart doctor finally explained how to optimize pain medication. Dosages should be adjusted so that the extended-release, systematic drugs soften most of the pain but don't make the patient dopey. Setting these levels, and those of breakthrough meds for pain surges, is a process of continual adjustment that needs to be regularly reassessed. On the back of a napkin, he depicted the point graphically. This was in essence what he drew:

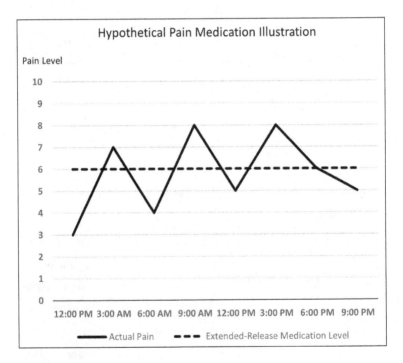

All of these drugs were taken in pill or transdermal patch form, although when Marcia was being given chemo or being hydrated as an outpatient, pain medication was given intravenously. During her final days when she couldn't swallow pills, she received high doses of Fentanyl by drip in the hospital, and Marcia was given a trigger to push through additional medication when needed. In the last few weeks, when we floated in the Smooth River, we finally got it right. Marcia transitioned comfortably.

Constipation and Diarrhea

Opioids are notorious for causing nausea and constipation, which add their own pain and discomfort. We all know that horrible cramped and bloated feeling of not being able to relieve ourselves as quickly as we would like. We bear the distension in stride, expecting the blockage to pass in due course. Now picture having that feeling all the time with no end in sight. A pancreatic cancer patient can be temporarily constipated like everyone else but the major source of discomfort for Marcia was the tumor's growth putting increasing pressure on her digestive tract. Normal-course constipation is far easier to manage.

Under her doctor's direction, Marcia took a number of meds for constipation and stool softening. One was Senokot-S, which combines the natural vegetable laxative ingredient of senna with a stool softener for relief of constipation. Senokot-S increases the muscle activity in the digestive system, causing waste material to be eliminated as stool. It is supposed to produce a stool between six and twelve hours after taking it. Sometimes, Marcia took regular Senokot and then Colace as a stool softener. Colace works by drawing in water from the small intestines to soften the feces. Other laxatives our doctor recommended were milk of magnesia and magnesium citrate, which is supposed to draw water into the gastrointestinal tract to help cause movement of the intestines.

Once Marcia was able to go, she was instructed to stop the laxatives and take MOVANTIK, a prescription drug to treat opioid-induced constipation. It's indicated for adults with chronic noncancer pain, but when you are in cancer world, many drugs are given off-label or repurposed. MOVANTIK was supposed to work for preventative maintenance purposes, to ward off sharp stretches of constipation.

For diarrhea, the advice was to follow the BRAT diet. BRAT stands for bananas, rice, applesauce, and toast—bland, starchy, low-fiber foods that have a binding effect in the digestive tract. Marcia was also prescribed Octreotide, which is used to control diarrhea and flushing caused by certain tumors and help with the cramping, bloating, and pain.

All of these medications have their indications and intended effects, but when cancer takes over your GI tract, nothing really works exactly as planned.

Dehydration and Orthostatic Hypotension (Low Blood Pressure)

Pancreatic cancer and chemo set off chains of different reactions. Nausea, reduced appetite, and fatigue follow. In Marcia's case, she often felt faint and needed to brace herself on furniture to keep from falling. She collapsed several times when outside the reach of something to lean on. With insufficient fluid and food intake, becoming dehydrated was an ongoing threat. Marcia tried to drink liquids throughout the day, experimenting with variations of Crystal Light, herbal teas, ginger ale, and homemade lemonade, but it was impossible to stay ahead of the mayhem.

Virtually all bodily functions depend on water. Water transports nutrients and oxygen, controls heart rate and blood pressure, regulates body temperature, protects our organs, and removes waste and toxins. Without sufficient water levels, you cannot survive.

Dehydration was especially dangerous for Marcia because it led to orthostatic hypotension, a dramatic falling of blood pressure when she stood. We learned the hard way about that when Marcia buckled during a walk along the Hudson River on September 26 (Day 23). It was quite scary. She grabbed a bench to keep from falling over, and I had to support her back to our car and make an emergency visit to the Suburban Cancer Center. Without this facility, we would have had to go to the emergency room of a hospital that didn't know us and start a new record, new account, new billings, and new medical relationships outside the ecosystem of our oncologist. They gave Marcia a liter or two of saline and, before discharging her, checked her blood pressure while lying down, sitting up, and then standing. We dodged a bullet, as dramatic drops in blood pressure can be life-threatening. We dodged another the very next day, when Marcia almost fainted again. So back we went to the cancer center for the same routine.

We had to go to the Suburban Cancer Center many times in the next few weeks, sometimes on a Saturday or Sunday, on an urgent basis. The center does not have overnight rooms or an ER per se, but it does have an "urgent care" clinic that is open during the weekends. When patients go there, they are supposed to call their main oncologist ahead of time to make an appointment or at least alert the facility in advance. Several times, due to emergencies, we had to make this call en route or just show up, apologizing for not calling in advance and asking for forgiveness.

Just like with pain management, where a plan that anticipates sharp pangs should be set up with extended-release medications early in the game, it would also seem prudent to schedule regular hydration sessions in between chemo rounds in an attempt to prevent perilous drops in fluid levels and blood pressure. Given the aggressiveness of Marcia's cancer, nothing could have stopped it, but that doesn't mean an organized plan couldn't be set up to manage problems that are highly predictable. Scheduling regular hydrations and other vital-sign check-ins should be integral to cancer care. We learned this on the fly as we sought to solidify the loose pieces of the cancer puzzle into a coherent mindset that became the Smooth River.

Eating, Digestion, and Nausea

Because a core function of the pancreas is to make enzymes that break down food and aid digestion, the chaos caused by the cancer and the chemo toxins rough up the digestive system. With enzyme production disrupted, it is hard to absorb and use fat and nutrients in food, resulting in diarrhea, cramping, bloating, and gas. Pancreatic enzyme pills are designed to help but are no match for the advancing cancer.

Weight loss is a common by-product of pancreatic cancer and chemo. But holding on to body mass isn't so simple when your appetite is wiped out by nausea and other symptoms. And then there are the cascading effects: weakness, fatigue, and loss of muscle tone. One's entire well-being is under siege.

What to eat became for us a function of trial and error. Textbook good foods included:

Fruits and Vegetables
▸ Blueberries
▸ Broccoli
▸ Oranges
▸ Kale
▸ Spinach

Easy-to-Digest, Protein-Rich Foods
▸ Eggs
▸ Nut butters
▸ Tofu
▸ Fish
▸ Poultry

Complex Carbohydrates for Energy
▸ Potatoes
▸ Beans
▸ Lentils
▸ Oatmeal
▸ Quinoa
▸ Brown rice

Healthy Fats
- Olive oil
- Nuts
- Avocados

Foods to avoid included the following, which are harder to digest:
- Red meat and processed meat
- Greasy, fatty, or fried foods
- Alcohol
- Sugar and refined carbohydrates

Top cancer care involves a comprehensive approach, including nutritionist consultations and adhering to best practices when it comes to food. Marcia and I took note of all the guidance and made good use of online and local health food stores and other retailers. We bought all the right things and tried all sorts of natural foods and supplements. But the reality is that you eat what you can. If Marcia had an urge for southern-fried chicken, steak, or french fries, her appetite became a source of temporary joy. Given the stakes, whatever she wanted to eat was fine. The big picture was to find rays of pleasure wherever we could. And if Marcia wanted to share a glass of wine to take the edge off, so be it. Enjoying food had the functional benefit of eating. In cancer world, sometimes any food is good food.

In the midst of uncertainty, we slipped into a lovely evening routine: dining by candlelight whenever Marcia felt like eating, sometimes with the news or a movie in the background, sometimes letting conversation flow without accompaniment. If she felt like going to a restaurant, the clouds parted and the sun lit us up even as we kept these outings short and sweet. We would bask in a fraction of normalcy. We would take what we could get.

As the cancer progressed, all meals became a challenge for Marcia, especially when food didn't taste good anymore and became associated with nausea and constipation. She felt pressure to eat to slow and hopefully reverse the shrinking of her body. Almost everyone encouraged her to eat more and break the empty-stomach/nausea/pain cycle. But no one could fully understand the biological turbulence continuing to build.

Before long, Marcia started throwing up everything, sometimes with blood. Often, she had an attack of dry heaves. This occurs when you attempt to vomit but can't. The airway closes while the diaphragm contracts, but nothing comes out. Retching is raw and painful. It was heartbreaking to see Marcia go through this ordeal. Medical personnel recommended that instead of meals Marcia eat like a bird, having small snacks throughout the day of whatever appealed to her.

Patients can feel isolated with everyone around them telling them what to do and offering them advice or prescriptions for this symptom or that. But if the fix was so easy, solutions would have been invented long ago. What became clear was that living in Marcia's skin took guts, which she already had and I had to develop. Seeing her in such discomfort with little I could do about it was a hard lesson to absorb.

Marcia rotated among various drinks, whatever was tolerable. Water often seemed tasteless and unsatisfying by itself, as necessary as hydration was. Her mainstays were ginger ale, sweetened iced tea, Crystal Light, Arnold Palmers (iced tea plus lemonade), and ginger-flavored hot tea. At times, she liked chicken matzo ball soup and bland pasta in butter sauce. Sometimes, she needed something cold, other times foods at room temperature or warm. Eating and drinking were work. It was upsetting to see her toil over basic bodily functions we just assume work automatically. During the two-day period when she took home the FOLFIRINOX ambulatory pump, ingesting anything cold could burn her throat, so we had to be extra careful to manage her temperature intake.

As suggested by an integrative medicine doctor, we prioritized high-impact foods—those that would help her gain weight, be nutritious, and not just temporarily fill her up. I purchased a blender to make her smoothies, but Marcia resisted and I returned it. Weeks later—after her inability to eat solid food became more pronounced and with the advice of a trainer/nutritionist—I bought another blender, this one being quicker and easier to use.

That was how I became a smoothie chef: I began to develop concoctions that Marcia came to love. For the key ingredient, I spent a good deal of time at health food and vitamin stores and online at Amazon.com, hunting down high-caloric protein powders. I was concerned that heavy-duty muscle milk powder would be too strong for her but finally came upon Naked Mass, a natural, vegan, weight-gain protein powder with over twelve hundred calories per serving. I was initially bummed out that it did not have any flavor, but that turned out to be a plus because I could customize the flavor as Marcia liked. A typical concoction included ice, water, a scoop or two of Naked Mass, chocolate syrup, bananas, and strawberries (which I bought fresh, cut up, and froze). Almost always, I snuck in almond butter, honey, and occasionally blackstrap molasses. Sometimes, Marcia wanted coffee ice cream in the mix. She tried all flavors of Ensure, Atkins, and BOOST but ended up liking the homemade smoothies best. The smoothies were the last thing resembling food that Marcia consumed. I brought them in an insulated tumbler every day when she was in the hospital, including her last week when I slept in a chair in her room. I woke up around 5:00 a.m. each day, drove home, checked the mail, showered, made the smoothie, and returned before she woke up.

Toward the end, it was obvious that Marcia had trouble holding anything down. Not eating wasn't her fault; the cancer and the chemo had been slowly decaying her system for months. When the end approaches, one's body needs less food and metabolism quiets to a whisper, unable to run the normal biological rhythms we all became accustomed to.

Anemia (Low Hemoglobin/Red Blood Cell Count)

On December 16 (Day 104), Marcia had her first bout of anemia: insufficient red blood cell and hemoglobin levels. Hemoglobin is an iron-rich protein that transports oxygen throughout the body, providing sustenance to our organs. Anemia is the result of not having enough healthy red blood cells or the existing cells not functioning properly. Cancer patients are especially prone to anemia for several reasons: the cancer can cause internal bleeding, treatments can suppress the bone marrow's production of red blood cells, autoimmune responses can destroy normal red blood cells, and disruptions in normal biological functions can also harm red blood cell activity.

Eating more iron-rich foods such as dark-green, leafy vegetables; sweet potatoes; prunes; raisins; beans; meat; and fish can help to avoid and treat anemia in some cases. But on December 16, our case was emergent and Marcia required an immediate blood transfusion. In medical speak, *emergent* means "arising suddenly and unexpectedly and calling for prompt or urgent action." During Marcia's 160 days of survival, we heard doctors and nurses use the term *emergent* so often that it regularly sloshed through our minds like choppy water lapping against a rocky shoreline. Surrounded by all things emergent, we became used to it. It was almost like we mentally tamed all things emergent to become part of our Smooth River. We didn't want anything to upset our peace. Marcia's life was too important.

Marcia's bout with anemia occurred, notably, a few days after the second treatment of Gem-Abraxane, the chemo she had begun after the first one, FOLFIRINOX, failed. Right before a hydration session on Day 104, Marcia became very weak and was about to fall. Being given saline hydration and a few units of blood helped to stabilize her. But the experience signified something far more ominous than a need for blood, as you will see.

Anxiety and Depression
Given the enormity of a cancer diagnosis, anxiety and depression are common among patients, especially the terminally ill.

It is worthwhile to be on the lookout for the signs of depression and to see a mental health professional early on. Most oncology departments offer their patients multifaceted services, including emotional health. We partook in them all: nutrition, physical and occupational therapy, integrative medicine, palliative care, and mental health services. Common signs of depression that may merit professional help include: a hopeless outlook; losing interest in activities that were previously enjoyable; sleep problems; material loss of energy; major changes in appetite and weight; mood swings; and suicidal thinking.

Fatigue, poor appetite, and sleep changes may masquerade as an emotional issue but could instead be side effects of cancer treatment that linger after treatment is over. Ask your oncologist about the possible causes of these symptoms and if depression may be a factor.

The prospect of dying is anxiety-ridden, made more so by pain episodes. Marcia found that having a mental health professional to talk with was valuable whether or not she was clinically depressed. She found it cathartic to talk things out with someone experienced with terminally ill patients. The therapist I found was in Northern Westchester, a thirty-minute drive from our house. We scheduled the sessions in the late afternoon so that we could have a quick dinner at new restaurants on the way home. The anxiety meds that were prescribed also helped lighten her unease and deflect pain.

For Marcia, airing concerns freely was vital in managing the strain of it all. Kept inside, negative thoughts and feelings can run amok without restraint. Prayer, meditation, nature walks, and other nourishing endeavors can bring some peace and perspective. But no matter how versatile your personal self-help tool kit may be, you should involve a team of family, friends, and professionals to help address the complex mental health aspects of serious illness. Whether or not you have clinical depression or other such condition, consulting an expert who can help sort things out and offer appropriate medication can make a huge difference in your quality of life.

16. Beyond the Protocols
(After Two Chemos Failed)

Man cannot discover new oceans
unless he has the courage to lose sight of the shore.
~André Gide

Our Smooth River thinking made space for the possibility—really, the probability—of the frontline chemos not working, that Marcia's pancreatic cancer being discovered after it had metastasized made it beyond the reach of reliable remedies. Yet we never lost our drive to do all that was reasonable to maintain Marcia's life on her terms. This included long-shot (actually moon-shot) approaches that were unconventional. But our eyes were always wide open. In our Smooth River world, scoping out something new and remaining active as long as Marcia could muster bathed us in satisfaction. Satisfaction that we were making the effort, taking prudent actions, imprinting our signatures on a plan. That was one way we reminded ourselves that life was bigger than that crazy thing taking over Marcia's body: it would not take over her mind.

The End of Chemo

From September 15 (Day 12) to November 11 (Day 69), Marcia had four rounds of FOLFIRINOX. As mentioned, the chemo involves four to five hours of infusion at a cancer center, plus forty to forty-six hours of additional chemo to be administered at home by way of an ambulatory pump strapped to her body. After many CA 19–9 pancreatic tumor marker blood tests and periodic CT scans to assess the effects of the chemo, it was determined that the FOLFIRINOX had not worked.

Plan B involved Gem-Abraxane, the other standard-of-care cocktail, the one that induces hair loss. Marcia was given Gem-Abraxane starting on November 25 (Day 83). But after the second treatment on December 5 (Day 93), the hope that the medicine could tame or even slow the cancer began to crumble. Given scheduling and other factors, including seeing how Marcia tolerated the new chemo, we were advised to take a week off and resume the third chemo session before the Christmas holiday.

However, on December 16 (Day 104), while at a regularly scheduled hydration session at Lawrence, Marcia's blood pressure fell to perilous levels, yet again. This is when anemia struck for the first time, reflecting an ominous turn requiring blood transfusions. A close friend had taken her to have the hydration that day while I took the train into the city for a rare meeting there. As soon as I heard what happened, I rushed to Bronxville to see Marcia and assess the situation.

We had become friendly with many of the caregivers in Lawrence's oncology suite and felt at home there. As Marcia was expected to stay overnight and get the transfusion the next day, our friend drove me to my car, which I had left at our local train station. An hour later, Marcia called to say that she had regained some strength and was able to come home and have the blood transfusion the following day. So I drove back to Lawrence and picked her up, and we spent a quiet night in our bed.

Anemia, in effect, put an end to chemo, which, in effect, put an end to conventional approaches. There was the slight chance that Marcia would recover somewhat to withstand more Gem-Abraxane infusions, but given the circumstances, that possibility was quickly dissolving. The stronger the cancer, the stronger the chemo. The stronger the chemo, the greater the toxicity running through your system. The cancer and the chemo were breaking down the vital mechanisms that enabled Marcia's body to function properly and remain alive.

With the two primary chemos having failed, we were left with no standard approaches to stop the inexorable onslaught. If our thinking had been derived from "ordinary mind" (i.e., prone to automatic, habitual reactions), we would then have been in a panicky freefall. But we had left behind ordinary mind months before. In our Smooth River mind, what might have been a nosedive felt more like a paraglide. We wanted Marcia's remaining time to be a gentle decline, first absorbing new insights from a high-elevation view of life, and then gradually descending to earth and eventually beneath it, if that was her destiny.

Marcia would collapse again, her blood pressure would plummet many times, and the cancer would rip into her stomach and cause internal bleeding, all signals that life's outer limits were closing in. Even though we were out of conventional medical options—there are so few, and they are so deficient—we had the resolve to move through interference of any kind, through any happenstance. We committed to not let anything taint our space. Our space—Marcia's fate—was going to be warm and beautiful, no matter what. The analgesic we had was bigger than medicine.

Investigational Meds

In mid-December 2019, around the time when the chemo options were disappearing, Marcia's wonderful second oncologist, Dr. C, asked the CEO of an emerging biotech company to provide Marcia with low-toxicity anticancer medication still in development with a differentiated method of action. This medication specifically targets cancer cells and disrupts their metabolism and defenses against the body's own immune system. Our oncologist cut through all sorts of red tape and on Day 104 arranged for us to receive the meds as part of a compassionate-use program. The doctor and the CEO worked out the dosages and, under their instructions, I gave Marcia subcutaneous shots every morning and evening, rotating locations on her stomach, thighs, and arms, in addition to her taking pills. As Marcia lost more weight, it became harder to find body fat on her stomach to pinch and make the injection. Several weeks later, when Marcia was in the hospital, we had to stop the regimen because the severe issues that had prompted her readmission took precedence over the investigational drug.

Given the aggressive nature of pancreatic cancer, its advancement in Marcia's body, and the experimental nature of the medication, the odds were slim that it would stop the onslaught and provide relief—even a miracle drug would have difficulty working at this late stage. But at least it provided some hope and therapeutic activity that Marcia and I could do together. We were grateful to Dr. C and the CEO for having tried.

Dog Dewormers

Across the street from my suburban office is a sandwich shop whose owner, Lee, I engage in friendly banter while waiting for my order to be made. For some reason, one day, I felt close enough to tell her about Marcia. As if on cue, she told me about her father, who also had stage 4 cancer and was being treated at MD Anderson Cancer Center in Houston, Texas. She then ripped off a check from her invoice pad and wrote down the name of someone she said I should look up. I stuffed the paper in my wallet and didn't think much of it.

A few weeks later, Lee reminded me to google the guy. His name was Joe Tippens, and he had an extraordinary cancer recovery story. He had been diagnosed with terminal lung cancer and was given three months to live and sent to hospice. Reading a blog post, Tippens connected with a veterinarian, who relayed a story about an accidental discovery that a dog deworming substance called Fenbendazole seemed to eradicate some cancers in mice. Fenbendazole is an antiworm compound used to treat hookworms, roundworms, and other gut parasites in dogs and other animals.

Tippens's world was contracting fast. Before the cancer, he had weighed 225 pounds, but the malignancy shrunk him down to 115. He was told he had a zero percent chance of survival. With nothing to lose, he gambled on the long shot and began taking the Fenbendazole. After three months of this offbeat regimen, his PET scan was cancer-free; it had been completely dark before starting the dog compound. Only when these test results came back did he tell his oncologist at MD Anderson about the Fenbendazole. "Joe, we can't explain it," the oncologist responded, "but you are kind of a sole data outlier right now."

Lee told me that if I shared this story with Marcia's oncologist, she would think I was nuts. But I did. True to the great oncologist she is, Dr. C was not only open to Marcia's trying this, she mentioned that antiparasitic drugs have been used for other cancer applications. So Dr. C's physician assistant phoned in the prescription to CVS.

Checking on the status of the prescription a few days later, I discovered a problem. The branded drug EMVERM that was prescribed was not covered by our insurance, and it would cost $29,000 out of pocket. So I went to three pet food shops in the area—Petco, PetSmart, and Pet Valu—in addition to Amazon.com to buy the compounds that Tippens had used. I bought packets in different strengths, each made for different-size dogs and each costing around $30. They come in a powder and are intended to be sprinkled on a dog's food. Tippens had gulped it down with water, but I didn't feel good about giving it that way to any human, let alone my wife.

Acting on my personal Law of Self-Interest—the person directly impacted by a problem has the highest motivation to solve it—I called CVS again on January 10 (Day 129) for help in getting the human form of it covered by our insurance. This time, I got a different pharmacist who mentioned that there was a generic alternative called albendazole that would be covered by our health plan and that it would be relatively cheap. So Dr. C worked out the dosing with the pharmacist, and the drug ended up costing nothing. Marcia initially was hesitant—the pills were so large they needed to be split with a pill cutter. But she kept going forward and began taking it. Our expectations were exceedingly low, but it did represent hope and effort.

We didn't have enough time to see if the albendazole would have worked, but, like with the investigational meds, we got the satisfaction of leaving no stone unturned and doing our best. Taking a dewormer might have only been symbolic. But sometimes, realities are so bleak, all you have are symbols.

Blackstrap Molasses

While Marcia and I were sitting in the cancer center waiting room at Lawrence Hospital for a hydration visit, I began to feel some tightening in my chest. I didn't think much of it because with so many things going on, I assumed it was just stress-related adrenaline coursing through my body. Still, I mentioned the sensation to one of the cancer nurses in the waiting room. Not wanting to take any chances and with the emergency department only steps away, she ushered me into the ED, and a few minutes later, I found myself on a stretcher wired up to vital-sign monitors like I have seen on Marcia countless times. It was a very vulnerable feeling, my wife suffering from advanced pancreatic cancer in one room and me in another being assessed for a heart attack. All of a sudden, my life flashed by like a windstorm, and I understood what Marcia must have been experiencing for months. For a few dreaded minutes, I was powerless to help Marcia, my family, and even myself. That was another reminder of how precious life is and how we must make each moment count.

It turned out that I was fine. As the medical team left the room, one of the nurses who knew of Marcia's cancer waited for everyone to leave to speak to me privately. With an endearing eye and open heart, she leaned over my stretcher to impart some wisdom she had learned growing up in the Caribbean. She told me that blackstrap molasses had been known to have anticancer properties due to its nutrient-rich content. It contains iron, zinc, selenium, magnesium, and potassium, the majority of the vitamin B complex, and high concentrations of amino acids and linoleic acid, a lipid thought to have an antitumor effect. Apparently, cancer was rare among sugarcane plantation workers who regularly consumed blackstrap molasses.

Although I knew this viscous sugarcane product had no rigorous clinical grounding to kill cancer, we were down to scraping the bottom of the barrel for a long-shot antidote, and it felt good to hunt it down and try it out. It also felt good that a nurse who had never met Marcia cared enough to lend a hand.

As it turned out, blackstrap molasses was hard for Marcia to sip down, but she didn't notice that I sometimes spiked her smoothies with it. Toward the end, I confessed to some of the goodies I had mixed into her smoothies. She just gave me one of her trademark smiles, one to express deep thanks for caring and trying.

17. Making Our Home Safe and Patient-Friendly

Home is where the heart can laugh without shyness. Home is where the heart's tears can dry at their own pace.

~Vernon Baker

As we were about to leave an appointment with Dr. C at NY-Presbyterian on Thursday, January 16 (Day 135)—the second chemo having failed about thirty days earlier—one of the doctors on her team asked Marcia about her stool. The question seemed an afterthought, one that might easily have gone unmentioned. Yet this aside turned out to be pivotal in defining Marcia's remaining time. Marcia responded that her stool seemed a little reddish, but she wasn't sure. This was a possible indicator of internal bleeding, a potentially big problem.

To find the source of the bleeding, an endoscopy was needed, but Dr. C was concerned that Marcia would have to wait too long to get scheduled for the procedure at

NY-Presbyterian, and if the tumor was the cause and she needed to be admitted, NY-Presbyterian might not have an available room. So she recommended we go to Lawrence. No big deal. Arrangements were made with our Lawrence friends to expect us and assess the cause of the bleeding. When we arrived at Lawrence thirty minutes later, Marcia was swept through the reception area, quickly admitted, and scheduled to see the gastroenterologists. Her room was on the special new wing dedicated to cancer patients, 4 North. That was our first time in this comfortable and well-organized inpatient space. It would not be our last.

Because the internal bleed appeared to be a slow one and apparently did not represent an immediate threat, the GIs did not perform an endoscopy during the first few days that Marcia was at Lawrence. After I left her room to return home for the night on Saturday, January 18 (Day 137), a nurse from Lawrence called to say that a room had opened up at NY-Presbyterian and an ambulance was picking up Marcia within the hour to take her there. We didn't even know that this was part of the plan. So around 11:00 p.m., I put some clothes into a backpack and Ubered to Lawrence so I could accompany Marcia in the ambulance.

Other than it being pretty late at night and Marcia being strapped to a stretcher and hooked up to vital-sign equipment, the short ride down to Manhattan was uneventful (save for bumping over moguls on the FDR Drive). Yet Marcia and I knew we were entering new territory, bringing us closer to the end. There were few windows in the ambulance, so I couldn't see out. When we finally stopped and the doors swung open,

I expected to see the emergency department entrance on the street level with glass sliding doors and clear signage for walk-in patients. Instead, we entered a brightly lit pocket of interior space that seemed like a movie set of the Bat Cave with blinding floodlights and directors barking instructions. The floodlights were the headlights of other EMS vehicles, and the directors were hospital staff coordinating ambulance traffic and patient entry. We were in the special underground EMS entrance of NY-Presbyterian, and it was now about 1:00 a.m. on Sunday, January 19 (Day 138).

The EMS workers wheeled Marcia in on the stretcher, weaving in and out of a complicated maze of corridors, bypassing other patient-filled stretchers, and heading up the internal elevators to the wing where cancer patients stay. Even at 1:00 a.m. on a Sunday morning, the place was swarming with activity. The central nurses' station looked like the control room at NASA during a space flight but with far more hand and body movement. How did so many people—getting up and down, jumping from one station to another, speaking on the phone and to one another, logging on to desktop and mobile cart computers, checking remote monitors, jotting down data on clipboards—know what to do? The commotion was a jolting scene to witness in the middle of the night when all you want is a clean, comfortable, and composed room for your vulnerable and declining wife. Yet all that human activity was, in fact, very orderly. What I witnessed was the efficient choreography of a major medical center, with each professional tending to his or her function and patient. Everyone had a purpose and was focused on improving lives, one at a time.

After lacing through a narrow hallway, Marcia was finally wheeled into a long and narrow room. It was a double, with a curtain separating one patient from the other. Thankfully, no one was there at the time, and Marcia got the side of the room next to the window, with a view of the East River and the promise of morning sunrises. This turned out to be Marcia's home for the next eight days as teams of doctors, nurses, and therapists tethering groups of residents floated in and out to determine the source of the bleeding, otherwise assess her condition, and determine a plan forward. At about 2:00 a.m., with Marcia tired but settled in good hands, I took an Uber home to get some sleep, there being no reasonable way to do so at the hospital. I was very aware that I had to pace and take care of myself so I could be clearheaded and "on" for Marcia.

In conducting the endoscopy, the best hope would be that the bleeding was due to a stomach ulcer that could be cauterized or clamped off and not the tearing of the stomach lining caused by the pancreatic tumor ripping into it. But, as expected, the cancer was indeed the culprit. The endoscopy revealed that the pancreatic tumor was growing into Marcia's abdominal lining and invading her stomach, an outcome presaged by the original CT scan on September 3 (Day 0).

The issue became what to do about the internal bleeding, given Marcia's state. An answer came from the rad-oncs (radiology oncologists) who frequently stopped into Marcia's hospital room. After conferring with one another, the rad-oncs at NY-Presbyterian and Lawrence recommended a limited palliative radiation course in an attempt to stem the internal bleeding and create some separation between the pancreatic tumor and the stomach and thereby alleviate pain. Both teams determined that it would be preferable to do the treatments in Bronxville because they could be done on an outpatient basis and Lawrence was less than fifteen minutes from our home.

Even though chemo had effectively ended by Day 105, leaving us at the cancer's mercy, we still hoped Marcia would have weeks or maybe a month or two longer and that we could fulfill her wish to spend her remaining time at our home. While she was still at NY-Presbyterian as the source of the internal bleeding was being investigated and a treatment plan developed (Days 138–145), I began to arrange for her discharge. I wanted to make our home safe and comfortable without turning it into an ICU, which Marcia did not want. No matter how disabled she was, she gravitated to clean lines and order. Our bedroom would remain a bedroom.

The first thing I scoped out was a handicapped stair lift, but it needed to be low profile and as inobtrusive as possible without sacrificing function. I called several stair-lift vendors until I found one who understood our needs and could perform the installation at night after I came back from Marcia's bedside in Manhattan. I believed that the cost would be covered by insurance, but that would be determined after the fact. I was now in a race to get everything ready as soon as I could to make sure that when Marcia was discharged she would be able to get up and down the stairs and otherwise get around the two or three rooms she would live in. She could no longer slide down the stairs on her rear using her backward crab walk technique, which she had mastered weeks before, or even walk anywhere without some support.

Being pressed for time and needing professional help, I asked the stair-lift vendor if he knew of any specialists who could help with other safety measures. Sure enough, the vendor recommended a military veteran expert in home safety equipment. He, too, came over in short order and, with me, simulated each of Marcia's expected physical movements and needs by slowly walking through what her routines would be. He installed grab bars and a handheld showerhead in her shower so that I or a home health aide would be able to wash her while she sat on a shower seat. He also recommended nonskid bathroom mats, a higher toilet seat, and a commode. I got all of that, plus several handheld basins for Marcia to throw up in, an ongoing problem that had erupted with little notice. I also ordered a lightweight, portable patient transport chair; a foldable walker to help Marcia move around on her own and get some exercise; and a gel cushion for the toilet seat. Because Marcia had lost so much weight, she didn't have enough natural body mass under her, so sitting on a hard surface for long periods was uncomfortable.

On Sunday, January 26 (Day 145), Marcia was discharged after NY-Presbyterian was satisfied that our home was properly set up for her and she was well enough to leave. I drove her home in my car, and our older son met us when we arrived to help out.

Things worked out pretty smoothly when we got home. The stair lift operated like a dream. It was quiet, compact, and easy to operate. With it, Marcia was able to make it up and down our stairs and, with my or an aide's assistance, retreat in peace to our den to read or watch a movie or settle into our bedroom. Late that afternoon, she took her first real shower in days. I gave her a quick lesson on the grab bars and the handheld showerhead, then turned on the water and helped her onto the shower seat. I undressed and joined her inside to gently wash her, shampoo her hair, and massage her scalp with conditioner.

I then left her in the steam to sit by herself to just be, making the experience more than a practical body wash. That was part of appreciating every moment and valuing the human body and respecting the human being. Maybe Marcia's love of water and her wish, at times, to ponder things on her own alone heightened a shower into a more spiritual cleanse. When she got out, I gave her a present: a special head towel that served as a quick-dry turban.

I helped her move to her makeup chair so I could have the pleasure of drying her hair, a task that over the months had taken on an almost sacred connection for us both. She was now purified, comfortable, and relieved to be home.

The last challenge of the night was our bed. We knew our regular mattress was high off the ground and she might have difficulty getting in and out and propping herself into the more upright position that reduced her stomach pain. But the nurses at NY-Presbyterian thought we might try our own bed first before renting a hospital bed. We quickly found out that ours was inadequate; it didn't allow Marcia to elevate the top part of the bed so she could sit up and sleep a bit inclined. The next day, Monday, January 27 (Day 146), I brought in a rented hospital bed. With that and the skilled nursing profession-als scheduled to enter the picture, we incorporated medical functionality into our bedroom, retaining Marcia-like decor. The orchid on her night table made everything right.

That Monday was a big day. Nurses from three different services were coming to interview Marcia to see if her condition qualified for home-care services—even though for the past two weeks, her condition had been so severe she had needed to be hospitalized. The first nurse was from the home-care company to qualify Marcia for an aide; the second, from Visiting Nurse Services of Westchester to approve skilled nursing visits; and the third, from our long-term care insurance carrier.

Monday was also the first day that we brought in a home aide. Until Day 145, Marcia's only aide outside of the hospital was me—reflecting how much she had declined in the past ten days or so. Home care provides nonskilled aides to help with everyday activities like showering, going to the bathroom, dressing, meal preparation, household tasks, moving around the house, transportation, and companionship. The aide an agency sends over is chosen to meet certain personality and other criteria as described by the client, but in actuality, it's a bit hit-and-miss in terms of whether the aide will have good chemistry with the patient (which often has nothing to do with the aide's technical abilities). The agency is more than happy to switch out aides until a good fit is obtained.

The first aide the agency sent over Monday and Tuesday (Days 146–147), for six hours each day, was nice enough, but there was some awkwardness, as Marcia wanted to move downstairs and then be alone in the den to read or watch Netflix. She needed the aide sparingly and wanted to get adjusted to the presence of a person whose key function was helping her move around and do her business in the bathroom. Marcia didn't want to feel obliged to entertain the aide or make small talk.

The skilled nursing agency was to provide a nurse to visit twice weekly for an hour to check Marcia's vitals, monitor her medications, see how she moved around, and speak with her about symptoms, medication, side effects, mobility, her emotional state, and other medical questions, including the process of dying. The skilled nursing service would also arrange for a nutritionist and an occupational therapist to visit, encircling us with what seemed like all the medical care one might need . . . except that which provides for survival.

On the third day home, Wednesday, January 29 (Day 148), the home agency assigned a new aide who was a better fit for Marcia. Her real needs were help with bodily functions, and although I helped her with these, Marcia now opted for a semblance of privacy by having the aide perform these intimate tasks during her six-hour shift. (Marcia and I had decided on the duration of the shift and, after an initial trial period, planned to lengthen it.) The new aide was 100 percent comfortable helping Marcia with basic needs without forcing conversation, and her easy manner allowed the two of them to share moments of levity and laughter.

It certainly seemed that we were well on our way to making our home Marcia's last stop, a place of serene Smooth River calm. Yet another emergent event quickly changed those plans. Our home time lasted only four days. In the afternoon of Thursday, January 30 (Day 149), I took Marcia and the new aide to Lawrence Hospital for a simulation of the palliative radiation that would be performed the following Monday.

Helping Marcia move up and down the stairs with the stair lift, ambulate to the front door with the walker, get to and from the car with the patient transport, drive to and from the hospital, and navigate the various stations within the hospital went like clockwork. All the painstaking preparation and careful measures to comfort and move Marcia worked like a charm.

But a few hours later, the charm lost its power, and things started to crumble. Around 7:00 p.m. that Thursday, we had to call an ambulance for the first time, for Marcia had collapsed. I was with her, helping her to our bathroom. She had dangerously low hemoglobin and blood pressure levels again. When we called the voluntary ambulance service, we made sure that they would bring us to our second home, Lawrence Hospital; most ambulances, when summoned, are often required to transport patients to the nearest hospital, which in our case was obviously not appropriate nor, thankfully, necessary.

All geared up in rescue uniforms and boots, the EMS workers made their way up the stairs, into our bedroom, and then to our bathroom where Marcia was lying on the floor. Like they were handling a butterfly, they gently moved her out of the bathroom, down the stair lift, onto a stretcher, and into the ambulance. My younger son and I went, too, holding Marcia's hands as respiratory equipment was hooked up to her face. In the slight fray, our screen door was flung off its hinges and flopped precariously in the dark, windy night, ready to fly away. No issue for the EMS team. Like they did with Marcia, they stabilized the door, temporarily securing it, and then accompanied Marcia, me, and our son into the ambulance. The next day, I called a screen door company to repair ours, and when the gentleman finished, he refused compensation. He did it out of kindness. The pleasure of helping us was enough.

When walking around Bronxville during one of Marcia's stays at Lawrence, my son and I unexpectedly passed his store. I went in to thank him, only to meet his wife, who was tending to customers on her own. It then came to me how to express our gratitude for helping us during an hour of need. I bought them a gift certificate to a Broadway show. They saw *To Kill a Mockingbird*. It turns out it was one of the last performances before the coronavirus pandemic shut down Broadway.

18. Room 413:
Our Final Home

I'm not afraid of death. I'm going home.

~Patrick Swayze

Things started to unravel quickly in mid-December (around Day 100) after the second Gem-Abraxane chemo treatment when, as mentioned, Marcia became so weak that she needed a blood transfusion. This started the post-chemo phase, where there were no real remaining options, where we were in free float.

Around 9:00 a.m. on Friday, January 3 (Day 123), I took her blood pressure at home, and it was a comfortable 117/75. But two hours later, it dropped to 78/56, and Marcia collapsed on the way to our den, prompting another hospital admission. Two days of getting fluids and having her vitals monitored at Lawrence followed before she was discharged Sunday, January 5 (Day 125), but not before suffering severe bouts of pain in the eight to ten range. That was when the doctors introduced us to Fentanyl pain medication patches, and pain started to be addressed with the needed potency and systematic approach. An extended-release, synthetic opioid, Fentanyl is eighty to one hundred times stronger than morphine. Marcia was started at a low dosage (a 25-microgram, seventy-two-hour patch). In the coming days and weeks, the potency would increase by multiples.

Thursday, January 16 (Day 135), was the day that the internal bleeding was discovered, which resulted in ten days of hospital time at Lawrence and NY-Presbyterian. Now, on Thursday, January 30 (Day 149), after just four days at home and just ahead of the palliative radiation designed to stem internal bleeding and alleviate pain, we were back at Lawrence. Once again, Marcia's red blood cell and hemoglobin levels had dropped dramatically. Once again, the staff at Lawrence were waiting for us and preparing a room on 4 North. We were immediately admitted, transported onto the familiar corridor, and escorted into Room 413.

We knew that things had changed this time. We were now in the last phase.

Room 413

Room 413 is on the fourth-floor north wing devoted to cancer patients who need round-the-clock care. This is the wing where private, personal, delicate, and kindhearted care is practiced with a hospice sensitivity. This is where the best of health care is dispensed. This would be Marcia's peaceful last home.

Big-city hospitals like NY-Presbyterian are at the pinnacle of clinical care and technology. The doctors, nurses, technicians, and other personnel are highly skilled and experienced. But due to capacity issues and building architecture, during her stay, Marcia had to share a room. Even with the window view overlooking the East River, only a curtain separated her from another patient who arrived the following day and watched *Law & Order* incessantly at high volume. By their nature, major hospitals cater to large inflows of patients, attract top talent, and invest in state-of-the-art equipment. While we experienced remarkable care at NY-Presbyterian, infused with warmth and emotion, neither it nor the surrounding neighborhood made for a relaxing atmosphere for us, and as I commuted from Westchester, often in bumper-to-bumper traffic, I worried that the high-protein smoothies I made Marcia every morning would flatten and get warm.

4 North at Lawrence was different. Marcia's room had the comforts of a real bedroom. Plus, beyond the door, there were teams of NY-Presbyterian-affiliated caregivers and critical-care technology at our beck and call. All patient rooms were single-occupant, and each one had large windows. Most of the time, Room 410, just a few doors down, was set up as a patient lounge where my family met with doctors and other clinicians or otherwise hung out while Marcia was napping. Although part of a facility with nearly three hundred beds, 4 North felt intimate, unrushed, even tranquil. Originally built in 1909, the hospital maintains a coziness in perfect tune with the charming, well-manicured, turn-of-the-century village where it is located, Bronxville. While Marcia dozed off, all we had to do was open one of the hospital doors to enter a neighborhood that was a delight to walk around and discover a wide range of quaint shops and eateries.

Marcia's wish to spend her final days in our home wasn't so much about the location. It was more about being in a place that felt like Marcia, meaning clean, neat, well organized, warm, comfortable, and filled with love. She couldn't conceive of being anywhere else. Her mother, who had died more than ten years earlier, had spent her final days at Calvary Hospital, a deeply compassionate hospice facility. Calvary was feasible for us but a distant second choice to home because of its institutional feel. It wasn't ours, in that our only relationship to it would be a place to die. And Calvary followed strict hospice protocols that would not allow the low-threshold palliative procedures we planned.

On January 30 (Day 149), when Marcia, I, and our younger son were rushed by ambulance to Lawrence, we felt right at home in Room 413, Marcia having stayed at 4 North a few weeks earlier. After receiving intravenous fluids and another blood transfusion at the hospital, we still expected to be discharged to spend our final days at home. However, with palliative radiation sessions due to start on Monday, February 4 (Day 154), the hospital thought it prudent to keep Marcia as an inpatient through the weekend.

Final Invasive Procedures: The Palliative Balance

Now was the precise time when Marcia's final days attained sacred status. This was when her desire to create the peaceful final environment—the last bend of her Smooth River—took shape. This was when the term *Smooth River* found its most profound expression. Although it defined the entire period of illness, things were now moving fast, and we needed to share our shorthand code with the clinicians so they understood what we hoped to achieve.

I developed some reservations about the palliative radiation, not because it would be harmful but because I would hate for Marcia to die the day of the radiation or to do the procedure unnecessarily. The point of the radiation was to make things better for Marcia so she would have peace and calm in her final days. I expressed my concerns several times to the rad-oncs, and they assured me that, going forward, one day at a time was their best recommendation and a reasonable approach. In life, we cannot predict the future, but after careful consideration of all the factors, we can feel safe-harbored by making thoughtful decisions aided by experts. And that was what we did.

Then another shoe dropped. Over the weekend of February 1 (Day 151), Marcia's feet began to swell, raising alarms with the Lawrence team and making them swing into action within the confines of the Smooth River. They wanted to conduct an ultrasound to determine if the swelling was due to the buildup of water or something worse. It was worse. There were blood clots. This was another sign that the end was near. The problem was that the blood clots could easily dislodge, travel to her lungs, and cause a pulmonary embolism, likely to be fatal. One doctor advised that this would be a quick and painless way to go and that it would be perfectly fine to do nothing and let that happen. In fact, if Marcia had been under hospice care, nothing would have been done.

Somehow, dying from a pulmonary embolism didn't sound Smooth River; it sounded too abrupt and harsh. It was painful to think about, even if Marcia would pass painlessly without knowing it. The Lawrence doctors suggested another palliative option: to surgically implant an IVC filter into a large vein to act like an umbrella and catch the blood clots before they traveled to her lungs. We were assured that inserting the IVC filter was a mild, relatively simple intervention, and, while nothing was risk-free, it was a reasonable palliative step in keeping with Smooth River. This plan, too, felt good. It felt like us. Here, like we always did, we assessed the problem, grappled with available options, consulted experts, and contributed to a solution that fit our personality, with the advice of our medical team. We were still being proactive but this time taking limited palliative action, nothing extraordinary.

On Monday, February 3 (Day 153), the IVC filter was implanted, and the first round of radiation proceeded without incident. In both cases, Marcia was gently transferred back and forth from her hospital bed to a gurney so as not to jolt her. The staff intuitively understood the Smooth River we were now on and signaled so in their slow, deliberate motions and gentle care they took. Everyone knew the end was near. Room 413 was now holy space.

On Tuesday afternoon (Day 154), after her second radiation session, Marcia seemed so weak that continued radiation lost its purpose. The medical thicket cleared, the bends ended, and the rapids turned into ripples and then a placid float. We had reached the final stretch of the Smooth River, the luminal space between life and death. There was nothing more to do. We were very sad to be here, but relieved. We were now safe and protected. There would be no more medical interventions.

This was when heaven and earth became one, when we could see over the edge and savor Marcia's remaining time.

The DNR Balancing Act

This was also when we came to terms with the DNR, the do-not-resuscitate order. When Marcia was at NY-Presbyterian for internal bleeding, the hospital had asked us if she wanted such an order. A DNR instructs health-care providers not to perform cardiopulmonary resuscitation (CPR), use a ventilator, or take certain other measures if a patient's breathing or heart falters. Marcia and I had experienced the deaths of our parents, as well as those of other relatives and friends. We were aware of what it meant to be kept alive by artificial means or aggressive resuscitation action. To us, this represented harsh, unnatural treatment. While Marcia was at NY-Presbyterian—Days 138–145—we didn't know how long she would have, but, based on the advice of the medical staff, we believed she would be well enough to be discharged to go home.

Once a patient signs a DNR statement and it is logged into a patient's record, it serves as an absolute directive. After witnessing the standardization that is often necessary in health care, I became concerned that a categorical code might not cover all circumstances and might prevent action that could be helpful in extending Marcia's life with quality. I needed to learn more and discuss this with Marcia. For instance, there was the possibility of having to temporarily put her on a ventilator and then conferring with the doctors for a few minutes before removing it. The DNR directive would have been automatic and final. I thought it would be reasonable

for a loved one to make the decision, with the aid of doctors'
advice, rather than a computer notation that may not have
captured all the possibilities that might then exist.

On Day 154, that time had passed, and, given Marcia's
frail state, resuscitation would have been dangerous in and
of itself. Refraining from a DNR order was no longer part of
the program or Smooth River. The DNR now became natural.

Living on 4 North

The activity of the entire medical team, from the doctors, the
physician assistants, the nurses, and the nurse practitioners
to the facility staff, patient transport personnel, and the food
service people, was, once again, something to behold. There
were so many instruments in the orchestra, so much division
of labor, so many shift changes, so much teamwork. Watching
everyone make their rounds, congregate at the nurses' station,
huddle in the hall over a computer on a mobile cart, have their
meetings, and exchange observations during shift changes
was to be part of something very meaningful. Here was the
heartbeat of health care; the very best of cancer care. The
one-on-one personal attention they provided made us feel that
Marcia was their only patient. But that was the same way they
treated every patient, so much so that when Marcia needed
more pain medication, needed to be changed, or needed to
be moved on the bed, we didn't want to disturb them if they
were in the zone and tending to another patient.

During Marcia's final ten days, my sons, daughter-in-law,
and I also made Room 413 our home. We redecorated a bit to
better personalize the space, bringing in some family photos,

soft blankets, a fragrance diffuser, and, of course, an orchid. We just hung out in her room, sometimes talking, sometimes listening, sometimes reading, sometimes wandering around Bronxville or getting lunch while Marcia slept. I normally got to the hospital around 6:30 a.m. to speak to the night-shift nurse before she left and then, as dusk fell, had an early dinner at a small Italian bistro nearby. I returned around 6:00 p.m. to say good night to Marcia and speak to both the day and night nurses during the changeover before leaving around 7:00 p.m. While Marcia still had an appetite, I brought her favorite smoothie in the morning.

During the final week, I moved in and slept on a pullout chair in Room 413. Yes, I had promised Marcia to be by her side until the end. But Room 413 became my home, too, because I needed to be with her, to experience this intimate period with her. The closer we got to death, the more intense and beautiful life became. Within the pain and sorrow of this time, the air was filled with gratitude. Gratitude that we had met decades ago and bonded.

With everything material stripped away and life ebbing, I no longer needed much. At night, I wore a T-shirt, sweatpants, and flip-flops. The first night, I slept on the convertible chair using sheets and a blanket the hospital had provided. But they kept sliding off onto the floor because the chair was so narrow. So, the next morning before dawn, I ran home to grab a sleeping bag one of my sons must have last used at camp twenty-five years earlier. It likely was never cleaned, but no worries. The chair and sleeping bag became my nest, and I slept peacefully within two feet of Marcia in spiritual calm.

We had a flickering electric candle for atmosphere, and I played soft music, connecting a Bluetooth speaker to my phone, to take our minds to another time and place that gave us pleasure. If I was thirsty in the middle of the night, I walked past the nurses' station to the vending machine near the elevators to get vitaminwater. I felt so comfortable and complete that I joked that I would be selling our home and moving into Marcia's room. Weeks after Marcia passed, someone thought I had actually moved to Bronxville.

During the last week, Smooth River was shorthand not to move Marcia in the middle of the night or check her blood pressure if that would awaken or otherwise disturb her. The entire medical staff knew that it meant the natural and soothing flow to a peaceful end . . . and a new beginning.

Adding Hospice Care to Room 413

Now that we had moved into the final phase, having conducted the palliative interventions and with the IVC filter to trap blood clots installed, on February 5 (Day 155), we opened up to hospice care. We did so even though it forbids, among other things, blood transfusions, classifying them as interventional. Normally, a patient in hospice would have to be moved to a specialized facility like Calvary Hospital, only a few miles from Lawrence. But Lawrence arranged for another service to provide hospice care to Marcia right in Room 413, as she was so fragile by then that transporting her could have been dangerous. Marcia wanted to stay in Room 413 on the Smooth River. It had become our home and the Lawrence staff our extended family.

The hospice nurses could not have been more solicitous, a seamless extension of the Lawrence palliative care professionals. They optimized the pain medication, making it an intravenous drip and giving Marcia a hand trigger to provide a shot of relief when needed. The hospice staff was like a warm blanket, tucking us in and preparing us for the end.

Communicating with Family, Friends, and Colleagues

As Marcia was waning, we wished to strike the right chord with family, friends, and colleagues. As from the start, we wanted to be straightforward but gentle and compassionate. As best we could, we wanted to share that Marcia was nearing her journey's end, but also assure everyone we had not only accepted our reality, we were also going to make the best of the situation. In this way, we sought to preempt any disruption of our Smooth River atmosphere, and we wanted others to derive comfort from it themselves. We wanted everyone in the Smooth River with us and to be soothed by its calm, cleansing, and gently moving water.

I wrote this email eight days before Marcia passed, not knowing when that would be:

FROM: Richard S. Cohen
SENT: Monday, February 3, 2020 7:27 AM
SUBJECT: Marcia

Dear Friends,

Marcia is in the last phase and we don't know how long she will be with us. Could be days or weeks. Your thoughts and prayers surround and comfort us. But Marcia and I know that you and others are also wounded, and we share our comfort and embrace with you. You have been instrumental in Marcia's life, more than you will ever know. Although pancreatic cancer is a devastating disease, Marcia does not want to be seen as a tragedy. She had the ride of a lifetime at Rubenstein and otherwise lived a full life with family and friends. I draw strength from her ethos of calm, peace, unselfishness, and modesty but also efficiency, common sense, professionalism and clarity. I hope you too can find qualities in her as a source of strength.

We are in this together.

Warmly,
Richard

As the week progressed, we drew inward, but we still wanted to keep our circle abreast of her status. We were living day to day, finding intense meaning in each minute. It sounds strange that we didn't look at death as a scary fall into the unknown. We were just floating in a dimension of life that had a window into the hereafter. It seemed Marcia's desire for clarity had prepared us from the start for what was to follow. It was far from familiar, but nor was it foreign. It was just natural. And it felt right and good under the circumstances.

Marcia made it to Friday, February 7 (Day 157), and that night was Shabbat, the day of rest when we are supposed to transcend our daily routines and experience divine wonders. This seemed like a fitting moment to hold everyone dear to us in the bigger picture we had discovered. Like other emails, I crafted this with Marcia:

FROM: Richard S. Cohen
SENT: Friday, February 7, 2020 11:31 AM
SUBJECT: Marcia

All,

I now sleep in Marcia's hospital room and leave at 4:30 a.m. to go home, shower and take care of some things. When I came back at 7:00 a.m. today, Marcia smiled and said hi. The nurses said her increased alertness is because the pain meds have been upped and Marcia has more relief, now being under hospice care. This is the final smooth river we envisioned, and although this is a terrible disease, there is beauty and inspiration in experiencing Marcia's remaining glow. Marcia is giving us therapy and telling us she is at peace.

Marcia and I wish peace and healing to you all and others who you know who are ailing. We now see that healing is spiritual and intangible even if it is not physical.

It feels good to be together with you.

Warmly,
Richard

Religion and Pastoral Care

Marcia and I were deeply rooted in tradition, liberal Jewish values, and the continuation of the Jewish religion and lineage.

We were steeped in the Golden Rule—treat others the way you wish to be treated—and enjoyed close relationships with many people of different faiths and cultures. So when Lawrence's Christian chaplain stopped by to ask if my sons and I would like to speak with him, we welcomed his friendliness and compassion. He enabled us to talk neutrally and freely about Marcia and our situation. He understood that sometimes we needed private time together and sometimes we wanted the balm he softly provided. On Shabbat, he quietly delivered a "Shabbos in a box" kit that allowed Marcia and me to recite the Friday night prayers over candles, wine, and challah bread. From YouTube, I played Debbie Friedman's haunting musical rendition of "Mi Shebeirach," the Hebrew prayer for healing.

During the last few months and especially the last two weeks, I had been in regular contact with our rabbi. We knew he had been following Marcia's health and decline closely and would help us prepare for what was to come. Along the way, I emailed him pictures of Marcia's bedside hospital table, which so typified her. It had on it an orchid, something to drink, and some cologne. Clean, simple, straightforward, organized.

During that final week, he and I began discussing Marcia's funeral, knowing that in the Jewish tradition funerals take place within a day or two of death. I wanted to understand the funeral's content and logistics, hear his advice on the number of eulogies to plan for, and other facets of the service. Because of Marcia's wish for openness, she and I discussed who might speak. Our sons also had some thoughts. Actively involving our rabbi in the preparation helped all of us unify around the themes and ambiance we desired. He gave us peace of mind as we planned for this impossible, inevitable day that the ceremony and the burial would be in keeping with Marcia's personality.

Ice Chips—Signaling the End

When you are dying, you lose your appetite, your sense of taste, all dimensions of the food and drink that sustain life. By Day 150, Marcia had not wanted solid food for a week. In these last months of illness, eating was a challenge. For a while, my family and her doctors considered the possibility that nausea was cutting off her appetite and, if so, that it might be managed by medication. But Marcia's body was telling her otherwise. The cancer was destroying her digestive system, and her body was slowly winding down.

During her last days, Marcia wanted only ice chips, which is such a common occurrence among patients that there is an ice-chip machine near the 4 North nursing station. Sucking on ice chips requires minimal effort and provides some hydration and a sensation of coolness. We were so far down to life's basics that it gave my family pleasure when Marcia wanted some. She opened her mouth, and we were able to place some ice chips on her tongue. When she slowly let the ice melt in her mouth, barely being able to swirl it around, her eyes were telling me she was leaving and she was beginning to say goodbye. She just watched me cry. She couldn't. She didn't have the energy. I cried for us both.

I have a theory that when you near the end, you become so drained that departing no longer takes on the severity it did when you were feeling more vital. It's almost like two divergent lines on a graph converge: one, the reality that death is near, and the other, the patient's acceptance of it. The difficulty in coming to terms with absolute finality is left to the survivors. Based on what she had read, Marcia told me that at a certain point, she would be ready to leave and that I would have to understand that.

I do understand that on an intellectual level. Emotionally, I'm still trying to make sense of it all. But I'm not alone. We are still talking . . . in the sense of my picturing her grin and imagining what she would say when I need to sort things out. She is usually telling me to keep going forward, be decisive, and not overthink things or get stuck in minor details.

Making Marcia's Life a Blessing

While Marcia was at NY-Presbyterian (Days 138–145), I started thinking about how to memorialize her, not at all certain how much time she had left but knowing I needed to get prepared. Marcia was so modest that few outside her work life knew just how significantly she had impacted coworkers, clients, the press, and the public. To do her justice, I wanted to create a tasteful tribute website that not only described Marcia's life but also gave family, friends, and colleagues an outlet to express their grief and thoughts about her. I wanted to have the site ready by the funeral so that I could refer to it in my eulogy and well-wishers could post their thoughts when emotion flooded them.

I looked at various templates for dedicated tribute websites, but all of them, while relatively simple to implement and lovely in their own right, either had restrictions that weren't right for us or seemed to lock in users to their digital platform and templates. I searched further, googling *tribute websites* and *memorial websites*, and finally landed on *Edna Jonson*. Edna Jonson was a memorial template on www.wix.com, an easy-to-use website development platform designed for laymen to be used for any purpose. At first, it seemed daunting to organize an entire website and get it done quickly and tastefully. But after watching some instructional videos on YouTube, it seemed doable and provided a sense of freedom not to need paid experts for the design or setup. I also got plenty of help from an office mate of mine, and some of Marcia's colleagues left their office one afternoon to work on her bio, a source of pride for them. Marcia had worked at Rubenstein for more than forty-one years, and her experience was rich with detail that only they knew. Then I asked her colleagues and friends to post some photos of Marcia in Google Drive folders I had arranged online for them. A key feature of the site being the tribute page, I reached out to a few of Marcia's fans when the end was approaching so when people visited the site after she passed on, there would already be some postings for guidance and inspiration. Marcia's memorial website is www.marcia-horowitz.net, and it will remain a lasting residence in the cloud.

Preparing Marcia's memorial website while she was still alive involved a delicate balance. On the one hand, it helped prepare me emotionally for life without her and consolidated my thinking in terms of carrying Marcia's legacy forward. On the other, I wanted to live in the moment and stretch out my time with her. How much to involve Marcia in matters surrounding her passing was also part of that balance. As I sat beside her every day and slept near her bed every night, I weighed what she might want to hear and discuss and what might worry her. Her being open to talking about dying did not mean that all subjects could be broached indiscriminately.

The rule I adopted was to not discuss everything but rather to put myself in her shoes—knowing her sensitivities and values—and discuss everything that I thought she would benefit from. As she declined, I was more guarded but still open enough to let her know that I wasn't hiding things from her. That I was preparing a tribute website and that her colleagues and friends were effusively helping was something I thought would bring her some joy. I told her that throngs of people wanted to express their love for her, and this was a tangible way they could do that, do something, right now. The news evoked that soft, glowing smile that defined her.

The Edna Jonson template suggested a page listing causes that held meaning for her and where donations could be made in her memory. Following suit, on our website, I suggested some nonprofit organizations that were dear to Marcia. She and I discussed the specifics of several. As an outside public relations adviser, she had previously worked on several issues for the Museum of Jewish Heritage: A Living Memorial to the Holocaust and its board of directors. Marcia had a keen interest in the Holocaust as an intrinsic Jewish tragedy and its universal message impacting other minorities, demonstrating where hate and prejudice can lead if not replaced with knowledge and acceptance. In light of the circumstances, the museum was more than happy to help us create a special fund in Marcia's honor. It's called the Marcia Horowitz Special

Education Fund for Cross-Cultural Awareness. Marcia also suggested the Lustgarten Foundation, Let's Win! Pancreatic Cancer, and our small nonprofit, Marcia's Light Foundation, which we had set up months earlier.

As Marcia's life was fading, I was afraid that the intimate environment my family shared would shift to more public forums and that I would be consumed with activity once she passed. So, envisioning what was to come, I made preparations for the events to follow, like helping to design the funeral and the memorial website and making photo collage posters to place in our house during the shiva, the Jewish post-burial period when mourners receive well-wishers at their home. I wanted everything going forward to do Marcia justice but not worry about frayed edges or loose ends. With these matters taken care of, I could experience, with less distraction, my own grieving and that of my family and embrace and be embraced by those paying their respects.

Day 160

Nights in Room 413 were velvety, openhearted, and teary-eyed. I played soft Broadway show tunes, piano instrumentals I found on YouTube performed by Emile Pandolfi. In 1980, Marcia and I had met at a bar in the Hamptons as strangers "across a crowded room," so our wedding song was "Some Enchanted Evening." That is the last song and the title of Pandolfi's album. We would listen to it every night and sometimes during the day, dancing only with our eyes. Conversation became superfluous; we would stare at each other for minutes on end, flashing through our thirty-nine years together in silent reverence as we looked into each other's soul with an intimacy I had never experienced before.

On the night of February 9 (Day 159), with Broadway melodies softly serenading us, she motioned me over just before I slipped into my sleeping bag for the night. With plaintive eyes, she patiently stared at me in silence, studying my features. Mustering whatever was left of her inner energy, with breaths slow and shallow, she whispered, "I love you," each word riding on a labored exhale.

I didn't know it then, but those would be her last words. She was saying goodbye. I believe she knew that during her final few metabolic steps later that night I was only inches away.

When I woke at about 5:00 a.m. the next morning, February 10 (Day 160), I softly called out to Marcia to wish her good morning, not fully comprehending what had transpired the night before. There was no response. Repeated greetings failed too. Sometimes she took awhile to wake up, but this seemed different. A solemn rush of the inevitable swept through me; it was the turning point.

Trying to do what I had rehearsed in my mind I would do, I left the room to ask a nurse to come in and see if Marcia had expired. She felt Marcia's pulse and put her hand on Marcia's forehead and chest. With tears forming, she paused, gave me a sorrowful look, and nodded.

For weeks, I had been bracing for this moment with great trepidation. I was worried I would enter some dark, alternate universe. But that didn't happen. It didn't happen at all. This was Marcia, and I still wanted to be with her. I asked the nurse if I could spend a few minutes with her alone. I had broken so many fear barriers during Marcia's illness that I came to realize their fanciful nature. I flashed back to the first time I had stepped into the shower with her and she had said she was embarrassed to disrobe because she was so thin. But my fear didn't occur then because she was my wife and I wasn't going to let her feel alone or abnormal. So now, in Room 413, fear didn't come either. Only love did. For 160 days, Marcia had been preparing for this exact moment. So, shielded in safety, I leaned over to touch her and kiss her cheek. She was still somewhat warm and tasted a bit salty. Her passing had been peaceful and calm, exactly how Marcia had wanted it. A new phase of our relationship was just beginning. It felt very strange but organic and natural.

The nurse said it might take some time for a doctor to come to make Marcia's death official so she could be moved downstairs. She said it would be OK if I collected her personal effects and drove home to shower, take care of a few things, and return within an hour. When I returned to Lawrence, not knowing what to do, I asked if I could spend more private time with Marcia in Room 413 with the drapes drawn. I just wanted to be there. She didn't look too much different from when she had been sleeping. She looked so serene and beautiful. It was hard to believe all that she had accomplished. It was hard to believe what had happened to her.

It was exactly at this moment that the Smooth River revealed its timeless nature. All of a sudden, I realized that our approach was not something reserved only for Marcia's illness and care; it was a spirit, a frame of mind, a lens to see the world. The spirit hadn't died with her. It would continue to protect me and my family with Marcia's values and remind us of her smooth, calm, and comfortable ways. All of a sudden, I felt comforted and reassured, regaining Smooth River composure to thank everybody who had taken care of us. Steadied by familiar guideposts, I knew I would also be able to prepare our family for the funeral, the burial, the shiva, our bereavement, and beyond. I would often falter, but I was equipped to pass on the Smooth River to those surrounding us so that everyone would be comforted by its soothing waters.

Within hours, though, Smooth River met its first real-world challenge in the after-Marcia era. I soon learned that the approach would not always be an automatic thought pattern but often would need to be mindfully activated. Before Marcia passed, the Lawrence staff and I had made arrangements for all intravenous connections to be removed before she was transported to the funeral home. In the Jewish religion, a corpse is to be cared for and sanctified by specially qualified people who are part of a *chevra kadisha*, or Jewish burial society. There are ancient purification rituals called *tahara*, which involves washing the body; clothing it in simple shrouds of white pure muslin or linen garments; placing it in an unadorned coffin; and watching over it in an adjoining room until burial. These rituals reflect the holiness of the corpse and honor the departed.

Lawrence did remove the IV connections but not the subcu-taneous chemo port, which needed to be withdrawn surgically. While Marcia still lay in Lawrence's temperature-controlled morgue, the hospital said that the funeral home should remove the port because they had experience with taking out such artificial items. The funeral home, for its part, said that when they receive a Jewish corpse, they cede all responsibility to the *chevra kadisha* and do not touch the body. The *chevra kadisha* does remove bandages, intravenous tubes, and other "insults of life," but I didn't know if they would use a scalpel to take out a chemo port under the skin.

My old self might have gone a round or two in seeking to convince Lawrence to remove the port, but right then and there, like a gentle wind, Marcia swept through my mind, and I remembered the Smooth River switch. In the scheme of things, removing the port was a small-stuff detail. I would change my outlook to see the port not as an artificial implant but as a portal from her soul to the heavens and universe. It would remain as is, and we would move on. And with that, Marcia was moved to the funeral home to be purified.

19. Marcia's Wishes

**The purpose of life is not to be happy. It is to be useful,
to be honorable, to be compassionate, to have it make some
difference that you have lived and lived well.**
~Ralph Waldo Emerson

In December 2019, a palliative medicine doctor who was part of the NY-Presbyterian team gave us a copy of Five Wishes®, the directive I wrote about earlier that includes passages that speak to the personal, emotional, and spiritual needs of a patient and his or her family.

I had been carrying the pamphlet around in my backpack for weeks and pretty much forgot about it. But as the end was fast approaching, something caused me to pull it out in Room 413. I think I intuitively remembered that in addition to legal information, it also suggested wishes a dying patient may want to convey before he or she passes. While the pamphlet's suggestions did not exactly fit Marcia's circumstances, I saw deep meaning in this insightful effort for a patient to create a message that would outlast her. So during the final week—not knowing which breath would be her last—Marcia and I did what we had done so many times: we took a well-rooted precedent and molded our own version of it. Using the Five Wishes model, I asked Marcia what she wanted her survivors to know. Inspired by the number eight, which in the Jewish religion has spiritual significance, Marcia ironed out her Eight Wishes.

In preparing for the end, this was a text I sent our rabbi on February 9 (Day 159) and our ensuing exchanges:

From me:

Rabbi, we had another quality day even though Marcia's systems are weakening. Even though we cry, there are moments of beauty on the smooth river. We don't know timing but she's not in pain and it's therapeutic to listen to show tunes and just be in her room. Below are Marcia's wishes based on a template the palliative doctors gave us. If the boys don't want to mention them at the funeral, might you?

Marcia's Wishes

1. *I wish my family and friends to know that I love them. I wish my colleagues to know how gratifying they made my life.*
2. *I wish to be forgiven for times I may have hurt my family, friends, and others.*
3. *I wish to have my family, friends, and others know that I forgive them for when they may have hurt me.*
4. *I wish everyone to know that I have lived in peace and that I start my new journey in peace.*

5. *I wish to live on in happy memories, humor, and inspiration, not grief and sorrow.*

6. *I wish everyone to remember me as I was before I became ill.*

7. *I wish for my family, friends, and others to look at my passing as a time of personal growth.*

8. *I wish for my family, friends, and others to carry on with strength and a higher purpose and not to sweat the small stuff.*

Thank you for helping me carry out my wishes.

From the rabbi:

This is profound and inspiring. This is in every sense a reconstructed viddui or "confession." Asking for forgiveness and giving it freely. Imploring her loved ones to remember her in her vitality, to continue remembering her in your own loving deeds, and to send her on her journey with joy and acceptance.

From me:

Thank you for blessing her wishes. It's nice to know that Marcia's heart and authenticity are rooted in Jewish tradition, better yet "Reconstructed," personalized and kosher.

From the rabbi:

The most kosher of all.

Our love is with you today as you find the strength to make the necessary plans. Call any time.

Preparing final wishes enables the patient to communicate simply and concisely a lasting message, letting everyone know how he or she would like to be remembered. It challenges the patient to summarize fundamental values to be passed on. It distills swarms of mental activity into lucid points that define the patient and provide direction and inspiration for others. Final wishes, in effect, serve as a lasting testament for what a patient stands for, providing a channel to express thoughts that may have been long bottled up. Teasing them out is cleansing and helps to cohere loose-ended thoughts and emotions for everyone. Taking on this project and investing it with enduring meaning can help envelop the patient and his or her family in Smooth River satisfaction.

20. Making the Funeral, Burial, and Bereavement Holy

May her memory be a blessing.

~derived from the Book of Proverbs

I worried for weeks about crossing the threshold of Marcia's passing, exiting our private family haven, departing from the peaceful float we had at the end, and, most of all, not experiencing Marcia again alive. Now we would be surrounded by others, and there would be definitive actions to take—meet with the funeral home, select the casket, make burial arrangements, map out the funeral, finish up a eulogy befitting of Marcia, line up the other eulogists, and interact with a lot of people from the many different dimensions of our lives.

But just as my fear about Marcia's passing turned out to be unfounded, so were my concerns about being overwhelmed by the funeral events—I was broken and ripped raw but not paralyzed. Here again, Marcia's lucid, open, and unpretentious manner provided the guidance, protection, and confidence to go forward. Not only was there nothing to fear, but everyone was entirely supportive and was suffering in their own way. My family was surrounded by compassion, affirmation, and love. It was beautiful.

By discussing the topic of dying for months, Marcia had prepared me, and speaking with the rabbi almost daily for the past few weeks gave me the strength to do Marcia right, which also meant comforting others. This was the start of making her life a blessing.

The rabbi had stressed that the tenor and details of the funeral were entirely up to me and my family, but had known us for almost thirty years and understood that I needed his shoulder, guidance, and active collaboration. He mentioned I could choose some music. I instinctively thought of "Some Enchanted Evening" or our other mesmerizing Room 413 music, but upon reflection, I decided that would be too personal and emotional for me. Instead, my family chose Eric Clapton's "Tears in Heaven" because everyone would understand the multilayered significance—the love and pain Clapton felt in losing his son, that we all experience death, and that Marcia and all of us are part of a greater humanity that shares pain. We chose a particularly tender rendition that was performed at a funeral by a single vocalist and a guitarist and had it piped through our synagogue's sound system.

After the rabbi and the mellifluous cantor (his wife) blended the multitude of raw emotions in the room into a somber and inspirational atmosphere, I began my formal remarks. I wanted to have an intimate conversation with the hundreds who came to pay their respects. I wanted to open up and share what our entire experience was like, from the shock of the "cancer revelation," to Marcia's making harmony out of mayhem, to the many efforts to tame the storm and our adaptation to the ruthless inexorability of pancreatic cancer and how we made every day count within a context of composure and love, all the way to the peaceful end. After I tried to capture Marcia's many dimensions—how do you capture a life in a speech?—my elder son spoke, as did Marcia's boss (Steven Rubenstein), first cousin (who was like a sister to her), and representatives among her work colleagues and friends. All this took place in front of a loving audience reflecting the diverse relationships we had built over the years. There were many relatives and friends attending whom we hadn't seen in years, two busloads of Marcia's Rubenstein colleagues, and a rainbow of skin colors, religions, and cultures.

The hard part was still to come: after graveside prayers, the family and others cover the coffin with shoveled earth. Having family and friends, not paid strangers, fill the void is considered the final gesture of *kavod hamet*, respect for the departed. It means you have left nothing undone. The scraping sound of shovels lifting soil and rocks and dropping them with a thud onto a hard coffin is a haunting image of finality, even if fulfilling the task is a *mitzvah*, or good deed.

That scene evoked an absolute end, a solid door slamming shut forever. But strangely, I didn't feel this. My thoughts went back to the serenity of Room 413, and the void in the ground felt like that room on the Smooth River. Marcia's physicality was placed to rest here, but I realized that this ground was only symbolic. She was safe within me, within our boys, within others, wherever and whenever we sought to experience her, whether that means heaven, nature, a memory, or an imagined presence. She is now everywhere we make an effort to see her. So shoveling earth onto her coffin felt like I was covering her with a blanket and tucking her in for the night. It felt comfortable and right—that she would want things clean, neat, and complete, like hospital corners. Smooth River to the end.

After the rabbi said some prayers, a Muslim leader whispered something in his ear, which the rabbi invited him to share with everyone. He said that the rituals and beliefs practiced in Judaism were the same in Islam, as the Quran incorporates the Old Testament—"From dust you were created, to dust you will return." Marcia would have loved that at her gravesite a lesson in interfaith harmony was being conveyed.

The next step was to return to my home, where we prepared to receive the community for a multiday shiva so family, friends, and colleagues could join to express their own loss of Marcia and comfort us. It was therapeutic to bathe in reminiscences of Marcia and the magic she had brought us. Although we were all wounded, the prevalent expression was a soft smile. It reflected the warmth, wit, and humor she had left behind.

Every shiva evening, there was a brief ceremony of prayer and readings, including "My Hereafter" by Juanita De Long and "Epitaph" by Merrit Malloy. During ensuing discussions, I recounted our Smooth River philosophy, seeking to provide guidance in how to interpret Marcia's life and death.

A few days after the shiva ended, I sent family and friends the following email:

FROM: Richard S. Cohen
SENT: Friday, February 21, 2020 2:47 PM
SUBJECT: Marcia

Dear Family and Friends (please forward as appropriate),

Words cannot express the immense appreciation my family has for your and others' embrace of us during the last several months. As I had mentioned, given the intimate and peaceful environment we fostered—we called the 'Smooth River'—we were concerned about the public aspects of the funeral, the burial, and the shiva. We now see the genius in this entire process in reminding us of the tight knit community that supports us.

Today was the first day after shiva, and in the late afternoon I drove to the Hudson River to sit on a bench we made in Marcia's honor in an area where Marcia and I walked to gain perspective. Today, I intended to just ponder this whole experience and come to terms with Marcia, all of a sudden, not being here. I didn't realize that the Smooth River concept would carry forward in a very tangible sense. The Village of Tarrytown is creating a new memorial and honor bench area on a bluff overlooking the Hudson and Mario Cuomo Bridge, and Marcia's bench is the first one to be installed. Watching the sunset over the Hudson was breathtaking, combining the Smooth River, Marcia's Light, Marcia's wish to be remembered with happiness and in personal growth terms, and the readings to find her in nature and life. There was even a family playing in the area and inhaling the surroundings. It was a good first step.

Thanks so much.

Warmly,
Richard

21. Carrying Out Marcia's Legacy

Offer me no tribute of tears, no moments of sorrow.
Do not weep for me. Instead, live for me.
~Rabbinic tale

A s it was throughout Marcia's illness, Smooth River is a
metaphor for evoking warm, nourishing waters as a frame
of mind that guided our journey. It describes the clarity with
which Marcia took in the world for her entire life. Yes, there
were moments of great stress and frustration, and during
these times, Marcia would see the glass as half-empty. Life
is messy, and so is dying. But whatever was going on, Marcia
had a nesting instinct to return to simplicity, authenticity,
directness, and love. The imminence of life's end validated
and sharpened the utility of this basic impulse.

As mentioned, one of Marcia's wishes was for her survivors
to look at her passing as an opportunity for self-development.
We made the best of cancer's maw, of a predicament that
lacked clinical correctives. While we accepted death first as

a possibility, then as a probability, and then as an impending certainty, we did not romanticize it. We romanticized life. I remember the hypnotic trance Marcia would enter while absorbing the ordinary and making it extraordinary, like riding in a car or looking at a body of water or sitting at a table or listening to music or studying her family. Her senses became acute, as if witnessing people, places, and things for the first time, in awe of their intricacies and makeup. Everything appeared so vivid, with unfiltered intensity, with deep reverence, knowing these everyday intakes would soon go dark for her.

So part of fulfilling Marcia's wish to personally grow is a new appreciation of life and its unpredictable and fleeting nature. Of the value of other people and everyone's uniqueness. Of the ground beneath our feet. Of breathing and being. All of what we experience will disappear one day. And that day may occur for us or our loved ones sooner than we think. Smooth River opens up our senses to take in the full value of nature's bounty and how we conduct ourselves while we still can.

The structures we put in place during Marcia's illness live on. In the midst of the pandemic, in Israel, our friend Rahima organized programs sponsored by Marcia's Light, displaying the foundation's logo and a photo of Marcia. One was a COVID-19-safe food distribution to hundreds of disadvantaged Palestinian families, another a series of hands-on courses to teach Palestinian mothers computer skills to enable them to enter the workforce and teach their children so they could participate in digital education with their schools. At the end of each course, each woman received a certificate of completion from Marcia's Light Foundation. All the participants profusely thanked Rahima and Marcia's Light for opening up consequential doors for them. In the works are programs in Arab and Jewish schools to dispel stereotypes and promote engagement and learning about one another.

Other personal-touch programs are being planned to bring diverse people together and help those in need. In these, there are no politics, no red tape, no division. Just humans helping humans and the goodwill that develops when people join together—whatever their backgrounds—for the common good. Even now, I feel Marcia's warm smile at the concept of disadvantaged Muslims in Israel receiving sustenance from a small foundation in New York set up by a Jewish family to make her life a blessing.

In the United States, Marcia's Light organized several specially packaged lunches for the cancer care teams at Lawrence Hospital and NY-Presbyterian to express deep gratitude to the remarkable medical professionals who took care of Marcia. A multitude of other grassroots programs are being planned to bring people of different races, creeds, and backgrounds together so they may get to know one another personally, form relationships, and dissolve stereotypes and biases.

Likewise, the Marcia Horowitz Education Fund for Cross-Cultural Awareness set up at the New York City–based Museum of Jewish Heritage: A Living Memorial to the Holocaust is fulling Marcia's wish to embrace other disadvantaged groups, showcase their plight, and light up solutions for all those subjected to prejudice. In March 2021, with help from the fund, the museum hosted a talk with

Pulitzer Prize–winning author Isabel Wilkerson to discuss her bestselling book *Caste: The Origins of Our Discontents*, with Rabbi Angela Warnick Buchdahl, the first Asian American to be ordained as a cantor or rabbi in North America. The book explores artificial ranking systems used to subordinate and dehumanize Blacks, Jews, untouchables in India, and other groups. More than 3,500 people registered for the program, a museum record.

Among the other legacies we have developed are the benches. Since Marcia's passing, I've seen families picnicking on the bench in Tarrytown, children playing on it, lovers caressing on it, and outdoor weddings using it as part of the ceremony with the majestic Hudson River as a backdrop. Closer to home, the duck pond benches are seating for families feeding the ducks, bike riders taking a rest, friends stopping to chat, and me immersing in a reverie.

As I write this, gutted by my loss and pained by the multitude of lives taken or otherwise impacted by the coronavirus pandemic, I come back to the gleanings of the Smooth River. No matter where my mind wanders, I'm protected by its riverbanks, especially when I scrape against them, and am reminded to dust myself off, recalibrate my thinking, and rebalance my priorities. Sensations of Marcia surround me everywhere. I feel her in my sons, daughter-in-law, and our grandchildren; in our relatives and friends; in her colleagues; in the memorials, education funds, and nonprofits that bear her name; in the humanitarian projects conducted in her memory; and in how I mentally process things. I need only open myself to the goodness around me, the sweet spirit that was Marcia, by flicking on the mental switch that turns on the Smooth River and quiets down the motors of everyday life.

With all this, I think about winners and losers in the fight against cancer. And I wonder, *How could we ever be considered losers?* We won, even in the grip of cancer, because of our Smooth River approach and how we defined the experience. We won because Marcia's life was always bigger and remained far more encompassing than her medical condition.

And this is the case for everyone enmeshed in a serious medical situation or other predicament. The Smooth River is not a magic pill or quick fix to eliminate disorder. But it can be a more satisfying and productive approach to process a bad situation. It elevates us to a level above the chaos. It encourages us to see our lives as rich, worthy, and beautiful, no matter the disease or dilemma. Cancer, ALS, or heart disease may take us down, but they should not define us. They may end a physical life, but one's aura and ethos continue. It continues in others, as explained in the next chapter.

22. Life after Death

**How can the dead be truly dead when they still live
in the souls of those who are left behind?**
~Carson McCullers

Times may change, but now I belong at the cemetery. It's
my place for peace. It is where I heal. And, to my surprise,
it is where I learn and where I grow.

I used to be scared of cemeteries. It was an undefined, root-
less unease fed by a lifetime of imagery across horror movies,
books, and notions baked into us from childhood of what
death and the afterlife would be like. We are all subjected to
mythical, supernatural, and religious currents that seep into
our minds and instruct us how to think of a graveyard and
those buried there. Even without these influences, cemeteries
are wrapped in enigma because death is. It evokes a Pandora's
box of emotions, many imperceptible, that may be hard to
contain, make sense of, and control.

It's not that I thought cemeteries were haunted, although society does its best to summon uneasy spirits hovering in the air and under the surface. Superstitions prey on these apprehensions. And, of course, cemeteries can unleash a flood of sorrow, loss, and unsettled emotion.

But where I go is not the cemetery I had stuck in my mind. Where I go, my wife was laid to rest. After all, this isn't a movie, a book, or some whimsical, wispy mind game. This isn't about preprogrammed ideas or traditions. This is about my wife and her grave, her home. The imperatives of the moment put my anticipatory fears in their place, again exposing them as groundless.

Still, the urge to return to the cemetery did not hit me until weeks after the funeral and community condolence period, when the activity quiets down, people return to their everyday lives, and, despite the warm embrace of loved ones, the grieving face the loneliness alone. When I finally returned to the grounds that first time as a widower, I was amazed how at ease I was. When I finally found Marcia's site after getting lost among the many rows and columns of tombstones, I imagined her soft, embracing look; her vulnerabilities; her clarity; her calm; her wit; her humor; and the love she radiated. I pictured her smiling, glad to see me, and saying, "Don't be afraid, it's only me. I can no longer hold your hand, but our minds can still meet. It's OK." Her practicality eased my agita and opened my eyes to what was really before me. I came to realize that when you peel away all the elements layered onto a cemetery, you are left with some simple truths. Someone has died and is buried out of respect for the life he or she has led, out of respect for human life in general. I came to understand that the entire aura one ascribes to a cemetery is a reflection of who you are and how you see things. It can be eerie, or it can be loving. And, for folks like me, it can be a place for self-discovery.

After a few visits, I felt so at home that I brought books to read and just sat on a bench to listen to the birds and watch nature. Sometimes, I became so engrossed in my reading that I forgot where I was. Outside the gates, the surging COVID-19 crisis that had begun to grip and lock down our nation only weeks after Marcia had passed was threatening the safety of everyone everywhere. So many lives were being damaged and destroyed, but the cemetery remained a safe and protected space. It was a refuge for me.

It became so comfortable that I began strolling around "the neighborhood" to get a closer look at the design of monuments and to read the inscriptions written about others interred there. I imagined their lives and all those impacted by their passing. The snippets of words attempting to describe each life and the composition and shape of the monuments became so intriguing that often I just wandered into different sections organized by different communities and houses of worship. I've come a long way from being petrified of cemeteries. Now I enjoy exploring them as a sacred museum memorializing lost lives, departed dreams, and a history of humanity.

All of this inspired the following footstone:

Marcia Horowitz
JANUARY 7, 1952–FEBRUARY 10, 2020
The Essence of Goodness, Clarity and Love
Adored by Family, Friends and Colleagues
Her Smile Will Light Our Hearts Forever.

I have come to realize that cemeteries, like death, are part of life. We will all end up there. It's a good place to visit without having an event to attend or the pull to pay quick homage. I found it cathartic and fulfilling just to walk around and contemplate the existential puzzles that drive our time on earth and what we leave behind when we depart. I go there to have mental conversations with Marcia and evoke pictures of happy times together, to hear her urge me to progress and not to worry. She tends to me there, still giving me advice and hearing me out. I may enter the grounds feeling tightly wound and clog-headed, but I always leave loose, clear, and light.

It was during one of my visits that I came to witness life after death, without taking anything away from other beliefs and interpretations. What I discovered isn't anything spooky, supernatural, or devotional in nature. It isn't even mysterious. Swimming in the Smooth River, I discovered life after death is quite simple and straightforward. If we let them, the deceased keep on living through us. If we truly understand their character and actualize their lessons—not just mark their passing on a calendar, but live and breathe their bequests—they become part of us and we part of them.

My new journey, grief, is such a complicated, personal phenomenon. Everybody has a different experience. Unwittingly, the Smooth River provided me a tool kit to endure the pain of Marcia's loss, process the turbulence of emotions, and channel all these dimensions forward, creating the fertile ground in which to nourish the plantings she left behind.

With all the tools Marcia left me, embodied in our Smooth River thinking, I've evolved into a comfortable and creative, somewhat organic, and activist form of grief. Many people check in with me, but I also check in with them and others. I see my sons often, and my grandchildren, including Mara Sophia, who was born four months after Marcia passed. There have been COVID-19-safe meetups and outdoor meals. I love speaking about Marcia with people who knew her well, but with many friends, resuming our usual relationships and not discussing Marcia has its own rewards.

I've taken the collage posters made of Marcia, created some more, and put them up on walls around my house so that I can see and feel her presence more tangibly. I've talked with others about some promising plans for Marcia's Light Foundation and other nonprofit initiatives to be taken in her name. The Tarrytown bench has become something of a landmark, at least for me. I have met friends for picnic dinners there and am thrilled when strangers sit on the bench to watch the sunset or just to sit and talk. And now the bench has company: the Village of Tarrytown added another to memorialize a longtime valued employee.

There is no getting around it: losing Marcia has left a deep wound and a huge void. But I have no intention of entirely healing the wound or filling the void. I always want to feel the loss. Why? Because Smooth River thinking instructs me to caringly cultivate the loss as a stimulus for me to listen, learn, and grow. These are just some of the lessons I'm learning. Others follow.

23. Smooth River Lessons

Death ends a life, not a relationship.
~Mitch Albom

Marcia and I learned important lessons on the Smooth River. Hopefully, they can inspire readers to derive lessons based on their own circumstances. The following summary attempts to capture core elements of what we discovered, but it is not meant to be a stand-alone digest, given the nuance and context of our story. They are meant to be foundational guidelines, possibly springboards, to come up with your own Smooth River approach in a time of need.

1. **Your life is bigger than any condition. Take the hit and widen your perspective.** Whatever your problem, be it medical or another setback or calamity, seek to shock-absorb it by recognizing that your life is bigger than the problem. It may take awhile to come to terms with a jarring event, so be patient. In trying to do so,

imagine yourself as a third party and envision the advice you would give yourself. It is helpful to talk with a loved one, trusted friend, or professional. Resist habitual reactions, and instead be thoughtful and thorough in forming a response. Do not ignore realities, especially in the case of terminal illness when time is precious and can be invested with deep purpose and meaning. You have the ability to handle any predicament with a response of your choosing, even if it is only a new way of thinking or looking at the situation from a new perspective—through a Smooth River Lens. The key point is to recognize the value of your life, your remaining time, and, as harsh as any condition may be, remember that our lives should not be defined by the way we die, but by the entirety of the way we live.

2. **Avoid narrow societal thinking.** Do not fall into the rah-rah cheerleader trap of mechanically going to war with your disease. You may choose to use every weapon in the medical arsenal and be aggressive. But before making that choice, have your medical and personal teams go over the bigger picture and assess the pros and cons of each approach, the probabilities of success, your prognosis, the side effects, quality-of-life issues, and how you would like to live out your remaining time. Whatever you do, know that managing terminal illness is not a sport or battle, and there is no burden on you to do any one thing. This is the time to value yourself and think about the big picture, whatever happens. Even if

you die, you still win. Winning is having lived a good life, whatever its length.

3. **Understand your core values.** In deciding how to respond skillfully, dig deep to identify your core values, and don't get hung up on the expectations of others. Recognize what fundamentally drives *you*, the impact you want to make, and the legacies you want to leave behind. Scratch out some notes about how you can actualize those points, and over time, solidify them into a fluid plan and then action. Discuss them with people you trust. Let them help you and, in the process, help themselves by doing good for you.

4. **Set your Medical Plan.** Network with the best doctors you can find who specialize in your ailment. In selecting one, personal chemistry is important. Seek out a doctor who treats the whole patient, not just the medical condition. If your challenge is not medical, find an appropriate expert to help you address it. Do research, look up relevant organizations, seek out affinity groups, speak to other appropriate people, and otherwise get informed. Put everything on the table when meeting with doctors and other professionals. Discuss all aspects of your illness, all reasonable treatments, and the risks and prospects of each. Build a constructive rapport with your providers that encourages transparency and forthright conversation. If your plan involves treatment at a distant medical center, consider also finding a local

facility near you for such situations as emergencies and vital-sign assessments. Discuss all aspects of pain management, including the involvement of palliative medicine experts. With your medical team, keep balancing the relationship between extended-release meds to get ahead of the pain and immediate breakthrough ones to handle pain spikes.

5. **Set your Life Plan and make every moment count.** After understanding the parameters of your ailment and identifying your core values, design how you would like to conduct your remaining time and live out your values. Separate high-priority points from day-to-day hassles. Create space between your new, more enlightened, and directed self from your old one, the one who had more time and was more susceptible to getting stuck on the small stuff. Find silver linings and exquisite beauty around you. Set short- and longer-term goals that are reasonable. Spend time with family and friends without feeling obligated to entertain or meet the expectations of others. Find ways to harmonize disagreements by unifying around your best interests. Develop activities and projects that are meaningful to you. Think about commemorative actions to honor and give purpose to your remaining time. Envisage ways to carry on your legacy: physical dedications like a bench, a tree, or a garden; a playground and/or projects that help others; or giving the less fortunate tangible benefits and you the intangible rewards of doing good deeds and rising

above your condition. Consider forming a new non-profit organization; a special fund, a scholarship, or a sponsorship within an existing nonprofit (especially a small one where your imprint may be more indelible); a GoFundMe initiative; or another cause. Open your eyes to the miracles of simple pleasures. Take nothing for granted. Regard everything as a gift. Live in slow-motion wonder. It will all end one day. For all of us.

6. **Speak about everything. Leave nothing on the table.** Talk to your loved ones about the end of life if that is a possibility you face. If you need a professional's help, reach out to one to liberate yourself from the natural tendency to avoid difficult subjects and sweep them under the rug. If you are the caregiver, train yourself to become a great listener and put yourself in the patient's shoes. If you are a doctor, imagine yourself as the patient and his or her family and envision what you would like to know to plan for the end.

7. **Be an activist partner.** Keep logs, records, and notes. Delegate record-keeping and communications to a designated partner if that is appropriate or desirable. Don't assume the medical world knows everything that is going on in your life. Tell health-care professionals how you're currently feeling, what your capabilities are, what your worries are, and if you are encountering any problems eating, sleeping, walking, or otherwise performing everyday functions. Advise them

of lifestyle changes, current pain levels, and other symptoms you're experiencing. Have ready an up-to-date medication and side-effects list. Let the medical professionals know you are their partner in your health and well-being. Build rapport with and express appreciation for them. Doing so is not only kind, it facilitates more solicitous care.

8. **Define your own experience and comfort those who comfort you.** If you want private space and time, that is your prerogative. You come first, and those around you will understand that. It's OK to be friendly and diplomatic but frank and open about your needs with people who want to do things for you. You certainly may want company and the enjoyment of being with others without it being a burden on you. Assuming you have come to some terms with your condition, communicate your perspective to others. It will comfort and guide them. Just like in the broader culture, many people are uneasy discussing death and dying, and they don't want to say the wrong thing or do anything that will make you feel sad or uncomfortable. Cut them some slack, and make it easier for them to interact. Just be real, be friendly, and show your humanity.

9. **Memorialize final wishes and prepare legal documents.** Make the prospect of life's end a learning and growth experience. With a loved one's assistance, develop enduring wishes to convey to your survivors. Preparing

them can be cathartic and serve as a loving bridge to those surrounding you. They can convey forgiveness to those who harbor guilt, ask for forgiveness from those you may have offended, define how you would like to be remembered, and soothe and inspire mourners to live with higher purpose. Developing final wishes is a powerful project with lasting impact. Confer with professionals about wills, health-care proxies, living wills, insurance, and other legal matters.

10. **Grieve as an activist—a special word to loved ones.** Grief is deeply personal. Everyone's circumstances are different. There are certainly ups and downs and new revelations and insights learned along the way. There will be many triggers that mentally bring your loved one back to life, cause you to replay good times you had together, and evoke deep pain that he or she is gone. There will be sorrow and regrets for disagreements you had. All relationships involve peaks and valleys. Don't dwell on the downers. Tell the self-judge to take a hike. Reach out to grief counselors and others similarly situated when you need them, as many relatives and friends may not understand the swirl of emotions that are part of your new reality. To socialize and ease your way back into the flow, break the ice and reach out to friends. Don't sit by the phone and wait for them to contact you. If you are a friend or colleague, tell those in grief that you are thinking of them and are available for support and companionship. Remember

Albert Einstein's prescient words: "Life is like riding a bicycle. To keep your balance, you must keep moving." Loss leaves a deep wound. But it is one that you never want to heal entirely, as it will serve as an inspiration to make you more humble, caring, and reverential toward life. That may be the deepest form of appreciation you can give your loved one. Make their life and yours a blessing.

Epilogue

For life and death are one,
even as the river and the sea are one.
~Kahlil Gibran

February 12, 2020 was the day of Marcia's funeral. It was also the day the stock market reached an all-time high. A few weeks later, the coronavirus pandemic disrupted everything. Had Marcia survived a few more weeks into March, April, or May, we would not have been able to have an in-person funeral, burial, and other bracing, supportive gatherings. My family might not have been able to visit her in the hospital, and Marcia might have died alone.

When we look back at our experience, we are grateful for that bittersweet stroke of timing. Yet our hearts go out to the victims of COVID-19 and their families and everybody else impacted directly or indirectly. We look for the words to thank the tireless, selfless health-care workers; the incredible individuals who make, distribute, sell, and deliver our food and other supplies; and everyone else who contributes benevolently to our lives and provides us with a sense of safety.

I would like to think that some comfort, relief, and inspiration can be derived by seeing all turmoil and loss through a Smooth River wide-angle lens. Helping others is the purpose of this book.

Appendix 1:
Our Log (Condensed)

Date	Days After Diagnosis	Event	Comments
9/3/19	0	CT scan diagnosis	Stage 4 pancreatic cancer with metastases in liver and stomach lining
9/4/19	1	Endoscopy ultrasound (EUS); biopsy; genetic testing	Additional pancreatic cancer testing
9/11/19	8	First meeting with Dr. B, our oncologist	Hospital 1, Manhattan
9/15/19	12	Lab tests, chemo 1 FOLFIRINOX	Suburban Cancer Center (Westchester)
9/17/19	14	Pump disconnect	Suburban Cancer Center
9/26/19	23	Marcia near collapse, needed urgent hydration	Suburban Cancer Center–dangerously low BP
9/27/19	24	Marcia again near collapse, needed urgent hydration	Back to Suburban Cancer Center–dangerously low BP
10/2/19	29	Lab tests, met with Dr. B, chemo 2 FOLFIRINOX	Hospital 1–CA 19-9 tumor markers rising; chemo at Suburban Cancer Center
10/4/19	31	Pump disconnect	Suburban Cancer Center

DATE	DAYS AFTER DIAGNOSIS	EVENT	COMMENTS
10/6/19	33	Needed urgent hydration	Suburban Cancer Center–dangerously low BP
10/8/19	35	Consult with out-of-town oncologist	Suggested a lower dose of FOLFIRINOX
10/11/19	38	Dinner; first one at a restaurant	In White Plains, Greek restaurant, a welcome return to salmon, fries, and Chardonnay
10/12/19	39	Dinner, again at a restaurant	In Hastings, overlooking the Hudson. Pasta with vodka sauce.
10/14/19	41	Integrative medicine doctor, Hospital 1	Walk after eating; eat big-bang-for-the-buck foods. Took train to Manhattan.
10/16/19	43	Lab tests, Dr. B	Hospital 1; CA 19-9 results rising
10/16/19	43	Chemo 3 FOLFIRINOX	Suburban Cancer Center
10/18/19	45	Pump disconnect and hydration	Suburban Cancer Center
10/18/19	45	Spoke with Dr. B about FOLFIRINOX not stemming tumor growth; move up CT scan to confirm tumor status	Discussed other frontline chemo and phase 1 and 2 clinical trial drugs
10/19/19	46	Trainer	Low-impact exercises at our home
10/22/19	49	Trip to FL; walked throughout LGA and Tampa airports	Marcia had cereal and muffin on plane and early dinner of pasta with vodka sauce

Date	Days After Diagnosis	Event	Comments
10/23–10/24/19	50–51	Calls from FL house to business colleagues, friends, and family; visits with FL friends	Lunches at Panera Bread, sunset walks on Indian Rocks Beach, dolphin-watching, dinner out
10/25/19	52	Visit with FL friends	Flew to LGA. Marcia reiterated to Dr. B's assistant the need for time to review the upcoming CT scan and decide on next course–and not be crammed at the next session on 10/30/19 to immediately start the new chemo.
10/28/19	55	CT scan	Hospital 1
10/29/19	56	Spoke with patient advocate	Hospital 1
10/29/19	56	CT scan results	Mild progression. By phone, Dr. B recommended switching to Gem-Abraxane. Mentioned certain trials.
10/30/19	57	Met Dr. C, possible new oncologist	NY-Presbyterian
10/30/19	57	Lab tests; met with Dr. B; Chemo 4 FOLFIRINOX canceled	Considering switching oncologists and hospital, in addition to chemo regimens
10/30/19	57	Met with another possible new oncologist	Stressed supplemental, prophylactic hydrations
10/31/19	58	Scheduled hydration	Suburban Cancer Center
11/6/19	64	Having switched oncologists, liver biopsy for organoid testing conducted per Dr. C	NY-Presbyterian

Date	Days after Diagnosis	Event	Comments
11/8/19	66	Met oncologist at Lawrence Hospital in Bronxville, a NY-Presbyterian affiliate	Arranged for disconnects, interim hydrations, and urgent treatment at Lawrence
11/11/19	69	Chemo 4 FOLFIRINOX; started Dicyclomine anti-spasmodic drug	NY-Presbyterian
11/13/19	71	Pump disconnect	Lawrence Hospital
11/16/19	74	Second FL trip	Marcia needed wheelchairs through both airports; considerably weaker and more frequent bouts of pain than first trip; had to bring in dinner
11/18/19	76	Needed urgent hydration at Morton Plant Hospital, Clearwater, where we made contingency plans before we flew to FL	Marcia felt too nauseous and in too much pain, periodically, to leave house
11/19/19	77	Flew home	Marcia needed wheelchairs through both airports
11/20/19	78	Scheduled hydration	Lawrence
11/21/19	79	CT scan; tumor growing; FOLFIRINOX failed	NY-Presbyterian. Considering Gem-Abraxane chemo.
11/25/19	83	Chemo Gem-Abraxane 1 after soul searching about next steps, given Marcia's weakened state and hair loss being a likely side effect	NY-Presbyterian
11/26/19	84	Wig fitting	With friends

Date	Days After Diagnosis	Event	Comments
12/5/19	93	Chemo Gem-Abraxane 2	NY-Presbyterian. Discussed clinical trial medications and the human form of dog dewormers.
12/16/19	104	Investigational medication started; home-administered via subcutaneous shots	At scheduled hydration at Lawrence, Marcia grew faint and needed to collapse. Needed blood transfusion due to anemia, but gained enough strength to administer it the following day.
12/17/19	105	Anemia diagnosed at Lawrence; blood transfusion given for dangerously low hemoglobin and blood pressure levels	Hard to get into car; took wheelchair into Lawrence; bad pain at night after throwing up pizza
12/31/19	119	Scheduled hydration at Lawrence	Wanted cheese omelet for lunch; smoothie around 2:45 p.m.; chicken tandoori, iced tea, and smoothie for dinner; and two scoops of chocolate ice cream around 8:00 p.m.
1/3–1/5/20	122–124	On 1/3/20, blood pressure in early morning was 117/75 but by 11:00 a.m. dropped to 78/56 and Marcia collapsed; rushed to Lawrence ED	Admitted to Lawrence 4 North to monitor blood pressure, pain waves, and nausea. For orthostatic hypotension, prescribed Midodrine. Fentanyl started. Trouble getting blood out of port. Alteplase de-clogged it.
1/6/20	125	Oncology appointment with Dr. C, NY-Presbyterian	Blood in stool, hint of internal bleeding; advised to get endoscopy at Lawrence

DATE	DAYS AFTER DIAGNOSIS	EVENT	COMMENTS
1/16–1/19/20	135–138	Admitted to Lawrence via ED	GIs waited to conduct an endoscopy because internal bleeding was slow
1/19–1/26/20	138–145	Ambulance to NY-Presbyterian, arrived around 1:00 a.m.	Marcia got East River window view in double room. Often could not walk to bathroom, needed bedside commode. Hard to eat. Endoscopy confirmed internal bleeding caused by pancreatic tumor penetrating the stomach wall. Radiation oncologists at both hospitals recommend limited palliative radiation to create space between the tumor and stomach to stem the internal bleeding and relieve pain. Doctors ironed out balance between extended-release and breakthrough pain meds.
1/23–1/24/20	142–143	Stair lift, grab bars, and other safety devices installed at home	I set up home as final resting place and made it safe to enable discharge
1/26/20	145	Discharge from NY-Presbyterian	Used chair lift, grab bars, commodes, walker, transport. All worked well, enabling Marcia to get downstairs and move around the house.
1/27/20	146	Three nurse meetings with skilled nursing, home aide, and long-term care insurance companies	Got rental hospital bed. Marcia needed to sit upright in bed.

Date	Days after diagnosis	Event	Comments
1/30/20	149	Rad-onc radiation simulation for palliative radiation	At Lawrence, I drove Marcia and new home aide
1/30/20	149	EMS ambulance to Lawrence; extreme pain and dangerously low hemoglobin	Admitted to Room 413 on 4 North cancer patient wing
2/3/20	153	Adapting Five Wishes to make Marcia's Eight Wishes; preparing for the end	Making it Marcia's own. I moved into Room 413, sleeping on a futon chair.
2/4/20	154	Minimally invasive filter installed to trap blood clots to prevent causing embolism in lungs; first palliative radiation session	Inpatient in Room 413
2/4/20	154	Second palliative radiation session	Inpatient in Room 413
2/5/20	155	Jansen Hospice visits	Inpatient in Room 413
2/7/20	157	Stair lift taken out of house; Marcia never going home again	Shabbat prayers in Room 413. Discussed with rabbi funeral arrangements around Shabbat.
2/8–2/9/20	158–159	Tender family time in Room 413	Broadway instrumentals, soft conversations, getting Marcia ice chips
2/9/20	159	Last words to Marcia	Final conversation with our eyes
2/10/20	160	Passed in her sleep	Waking up in a chair by her side in Room 413. Saying goodbye across the divide.

Appendix 2:
Marcia's Booklist

This list of books Marcia read, along with other helpful books, is intended to assist those interested in learning more about cancer and infusing meaning into their lives and those of their loved ones. These and other resources are also posted at www.smoothriver.org.

Albom, Mitch. *Tuesdays with Morrie: An Old Man, A Young Man, and Life's Greatest Lesson.* Broadway Books, 1997.

Didion, Joan. *The Year of Magical Thinking.* Knopf, Borzoi Books, 2005.

Gawande, Atul. *Being Mortal: Medicine and What Matters in the End.* Metropolitan Books, 2014.

Kalanithi, Paul. *When Breath Becomes Air.* Random House, 2016.

Kübler-Ross, Elisabeth, MD. *On Death & Dying: What the Dying Have to Teach Doctors, Nurses, Clergy & Their Own Families.* Simon & Schuster, 1969.

Kushner, Harold S. *Living a Life That Matters.* Knopf, Borzoi Books, 2001.

Kushner, Harold S. *When Bad Things Happen to Good People.* Anchor Books, 1981.

Riggs, Nina. *The Bright Hour: A Memoir of Living and Dying.* Simon & Schuster, 2017.

Yip-Williams, Julie. *The Unwinding of the Miracle: A Memoir of Life, Death, and Everything That Comes After.* Random House, 2019.

Other Books

Butler, Katy. *The Art of Dying Well: A Practical Guide to a Good End of Life.* Scribner Books, 2019.

Kessler, David. *Finding Meaning: The Sixth Stage of Grief.* Simon & Schuster, 2019.

Kessler, David. *The Needs of the Dying: A Guide for Bringing Hope, Comfort, and Love to Life's Final Chapter.* HarperCollins, 1997.

Kramer, Kay and Herbert Kramer. *Conversations at Midnight: Coming to Terms with Dying and Death.* Avon Books, 1994.

Appendix 3:
Resources

The following list of resources is an abbreviated version of the more in-depth one posted on www.smoothriver. org, where organizations and resources dealing with many prevalent cancers and end-of-life matters are described.

General

- ‣ Cancer statistics (National Cancer Care Institute)—The nation's leader in cancer research
- ‣ American Cancer Society—A major source of funding, research, expert and patient information, and support for all cancers
- ‣ CancerCare—Professional oncology social workers providing free emotional and practical support for people with cancer, caregivers, loved ones, and the bereaved
- ‣ Patient Empowerment Network—A nonprofit whose mission is to fortify cancer patients and care partners with the knowledge and tools to boost their

confidence, put them in control of their health-care journey, and assist them in receiving the best, most personalized care available to ensure they have the best possible outcome

▸ Cancer Support Community/Gilda's Club—A global network of 175 locations hosting free support groups, educational lectures, and healthy-lifestyle workshops

Clinical Trials

▸ Clinicaltrials.gov (NIH: US National Library of Medicine)— Online resource that provides patients, their family members, health-care professionals, researchers, and the public with easy access to information on publicly and privately supported clinical studies on a wide range of diseases and conditions

Pancreatic Cancer

▸ Lustgarten Foundation—A leading funding and information source for the diagnosis, treatment, and prevention of pancreatic cancer.

▸ Pancreatic Cancer Action Network—A major resource network dedicated to fighting pancreatic cancer on all fronts: research, clinical initiatives, patient services, and advocacy.

▸ Let's Win! Pancreatic Cancer—Platform enabling doctors, scientists, and patients to share fast-breaking information about potentially life-saving pancreatic cancer treatments and clinical trials.

Advance Directives Resources

▸ Five Wishes®/Aging with Dignity—An advance directive to address personal, emotional, and spiritual issues in addition to meeting medical and legal criteria. With the help of the American Bar Association and end-of-life experts, and with support from The Robert Wood Johnson Foundation, Aging with Dignity developed the Five Wishes® program and advance directive document to be accessible, legal and easy-to-understand, with the goal of helping people discuss and record their wishes in a non-threatening, life-affirming way.

▸ National Institute on Aging/National Institutes of Health—U.S. Government agency that provides articles and other resources to help set one's affairs in order and plan for life's end.

Palliative Medicine and Hospice Resources

▸ American Academy of Hospice and Palliative Medicine—An organization of physicians and other medical professionals dedicated to the prevention and relief of patient and family suffering by providing education and clinical practice standards, fostering research, facilitating personal and professional development, and advocating for public policy.

▸ American Board of Hospice and Palliative Medicine—Promotes excellence in the care of all patients with advanced, progressive illness through the development of standards for training and practice in palliative medicine

Acknowledgments

The concept of this book sprang from repeated comments by doctors and nurses that the way Marcia and I handled her illness and decline was different. It was positive, uplifting, clearheaded, sober, and responsible when being lost was more the norm. Of course, during the storm of cancer, all we cared about was Marcia's survival and, failing that, a peaceful transition to the end. We used the term *Smooth River* regularly to describe how she wanted to be treated.

It was only after Marcia passed that several medical professionals encouraged me to share our experience in the hope of helping others similarly situated. At the suggestion of grief counselors from Jansen Hospice & Palliative Care and CancerCare, I joined curated private chat rooms for pancreatic cancer patients and their families, terminally ill patients, those in grief, and others suffering from serious disease or loss. There, the overwhelming emotional pain I witnessed made clear that the Smooth River perspective could resonate with many. From our own experience and some research, it also became obvious that Elisabeth Kübler-Ross's work—and that of palliative medicine and hospice professionals—is far from done: conventional norms still need to be changed to better understand and appreciate the dignity of dying and the realities of death as the inevitable end we all must confront.

I read so many fine memoirs and how-to books about death and dying but none that wove in all the personal, practical, and societal elements the way I had in mind to help others as a peer, one knowledgeable in health-care industry dynamics.

I first had in mind writing a white paper summarizing some points others could use. When I suggested this to my friend Mark Gompertz, who has worked in book publishing all his professional life, he asked, "What is a white paper?" I described it as an evidence-based piece that a health-care company prepares to describe a new product or technology, and it is sometimes used when clinical trial results are unavailable. Mark said, "No, no, write chapter headings and an outline of what a book would look like." Little did I know that the medical log I had meticulously prepared would serve as the bones and core content of this book.

Mark continued to guide me throughout the process, as did another friend, Susan Leon, whose career is also devoted to book editing and publishing. She was instrumental in the major structural formation, loving but pragmatic tone, blend of subject matter, twist of a phrase, and the glue and magic that makes a story connect with a wider audience.

Many other people provided real-world, unvarnished feedback regarding various elements that contributed to the final product. They include Dr. Jordan Berlin, Associate Director for Clinical Research, Ingram Professor of Cancer Research, and Professor of Medicine, Vanderbilt-Ingram Cancer Center; Dr. Eugene H. Hirsh, retired gastroenterologist affiliated with Emory St. Joseph's Hospital and retired Clinical Associate Professor of Medicine in Digestive Diseases at Emory University School of Medicine; Dr. Lynne Holden, Professor, Emergency Medicine, Vice-Chair, Diversity and Inclusion, and Attending Physician, Department of Emergency Medicine at Albert Einstein College of Medicine; and friends Edward Goldberg, Bill Doescher, Paula Wittlin, Catherine Simmons, and Richard M. Cohen, among others. Dr. Holden also provided an insightful, introspective physician's perspective in the Foreword, for which I am so grateful.

I would like to thank various well-known literary agents who encouraged me to go the independent publishing route because of the challenges involved in traditional publishing, especially for authors who are not famous. In the independent publishing realm, the author becomes the general contractor and has to sift through a maze of people and firms that perform one function or another, leaving it to the author to put together all the various puzzle pieces. My goal was to publish a book with rigor, outside criticism, quality, and solemnity, knowing I am addressing an audience of others touched by trauma and loss.

Several professionals from the Reedsy independent author ecosystem added design, editorial, and market perspectives. They include Anna Krusinski, Martin Beeny, and Alan Barnett, who not only designed the cover but helped with other elements. Significant final edits and perspective were provided by the Kirkus Editorial team (including Stephanie Summerhays, Jon Ford, and Christa Titus). The book layout and publication services were expertly conducted by Michele DeFilippo and Ronda Rawlins of 1106 Design and Bethany Brown of The Cadence Group. Corinne Moulder, Katy Schnack, and the other professionals at Smith Publicity rounded out the team of loving hands that interlocked to support this book and the causes it represents. Thank you to everyone for coaching me and helping make this book possible.

Finally, I give thanks to my family for their love, support, and partnership in keeping Marcia's spirit alive within us. And to Marcia, who still reminds me every day to tuck in the sheets, close my closet door, keep things straight . . . and to declutter and brush away the dust in order to see the big picture. Thank you for the Smooth River.

About the Author

Richard S. Cohen was by his wife Marcia's side when she was diagnosed on September 3, 2019, with stage 4 pancreatic cancer and woke up in her hospital room after she had exhaled her last breath 160 days later on February 10, 2020. Carrying out Marcia's wishes, he coordinated every step of her care, navigating medical resources at four different hospitals while also conferring with leading pancreatic oncologists elsewhere. Rooted in his love for his wife and bringing to bear decades of professional organizational skills, he exhaustively networked with leading professionals and researched the pancreatic cancer field, examining key resources, therapies, clinical trials, and data. He organized all aspects of Marcia's Medical Plan with her, her physicians and nurses, and an array of other personnel.

More importantly, he collaborated with Marcia in setting their Life Plan, the Smooth River, given her wishes for clarity, practicality, and relief from pain so that her final days could be filled with peace, dignity, and love. With

Marcia's aggressive cancer weakening her physical abilities and accelerating her end, Richard helped invest every day with meaning, being a gentle coach and giving texture and perspective to Marcia's cancer treatments and the associated pain, nausea, and other debilitations.

Trained as a corporate lawyer, Richard arranges mergers and acquisitions for medical technology companies. He is an expert in navigating complex transactions, developing grounded creative solutions, and managing many professionals and personalities during stressful conditions. All of these skills were put to work in finding sanctuary, beauty, humor, and spirituality within cancer's decay. Unencumbered by medical convention but having a deep respect for it and the clinicians who cared for her, Richard has translated Marcia's ethos into a creative, personalized, and inspiring approach for dealing with terminal illness.